T0372499

BREATHING OXYGEN, FREE FROM LONG COVID

It's time to incorporate Eastern and Western medicine for viruses and the lymphatic system.

HAROLD LEE

BALBOA.PRESS
A DIVISION OF HAY HOUSE

Balboa Press books may be ordered through booksellers or by contacting:

Balboa Press
A Division of Hay House
1663 Liberty Drive
Bloomington, IN 47403
www.balboapress.com
844-682-1282

Print information available on the last page.

ISBN: 979-8-7652-5477-6 (sc)
ISBN: 979-8-7652-5478-3 (e)

Balboa Press rev. date: 10/09/2024

This book is dedicated to my two daughters,
Suin Lee and Elizabeth Lee,
and their medical journey.

Contents

Preface

As the father of Western medicine, Hippocrates said, "Illness does not come upon us out of the blue. They develop from daily small sins against Nature. When enough sins accumulate, illnesses will suddenly appear."

After the pandemic, I seriously pondered this question: why do we go against nature without even realizing it? From our sleep patterns to our eating habits to our breathing, many of our actions are not natural. We unknowingly commit sins, consuming harmful ingredients in our food and beverages, as well as inhaling polluted air into our lungs. All of these factors accumulate, allowing the virus to silently creep up on us until it finally manifests. It becomes challenging to combat the virus once it is too late.

Viruses are smarter than you think. They mutate frequently against new vaccines, causing dynamic changes. However, human beings believe that vaccines are a cure-all, regardless of daily sins. It is not fair, so we should focus on fulfilling our basic requirement for immunity and seeking help from vaccines.

It touch me in virus invasion it add up in your inside invisible and unnoticed by medical test that is problem cause many people die

Dr. Lucy Gahan's book "Breaking Free from Long Covid" reveals the true story of her struggle with Covid, experiencing pain in her arms and legs, as well as a persistent feeling of low energy. She expressed, "I have symptoms in between with no cure, and I still have pain."

After the pandemic, nature urges us to incorporate both Eastern and Western medicine.

Why is it necessary for us to combine?

Is it simple to combine the micro approach from the western side with the macro approach from the eastern side in order to effectively combat the virus? viewing the cell-based systems differently from organ-based ones.

Addressing breathing issues is a top priority. Free oxygen must be provided, but we currently only receive the bare minimum, which is terrible.

The top cause of death in recent years is lung and colon cancer. I would say they are two sides of the same coin, like yin and yang, representing the same disease. Why?

How can I determine if I have a genetic predisposition to lung issues?

Do we know the DNA encoding, not by Western methods but by Eastern methods? I would say yes.

We also need more treatment options for invisible diseases. Each of us has a unique constitution and our own history of disease. Therefore, combining 3 to 4 options to combat these diseases can help us find more effective solutions.

Finally, never give up no matter how serious the situation is. There are many options available, even for combating a really bad virus, as long as it is done in a natural way and not against the laws of nature.

Chapter 1

Oxygen, Virus, Lymph Fluids

Hippocrates Galen and Huang Di Nei Jing

We first see a little history of eastern and western foundation

Father of Medicine Hippocrates and medical bible of eastern medicine

Hippocrates's accounts of surgery, specifically wounds and orthopedic injuries, were regarded as the most reliable until Aulus Cornelius Celsus (ca. 25 BCE-ca. 50 CE) emerged with his comprehensive compilation and summarization of medical theory and practice. Despite some erroneous beliefs, Hippocrates suggested trepanation as a means to alleviate pressure from head injuries, possessed knowledge on aligning clavicle fractures, and provided detailed descriptions on reducing dislocations and fixing long bone fractures.

Many of the wounds he encountered were incurred during battles. In fact, Hippocrates proclaimed that the only suitable training for a surgeon was to join an army and follow its endeavors.

Hippocrates offered numerous observations, recommendations, and diagnoses. He successfully recognized the physical indications of liver damage and dehydration. He described the occurrence of opposite-side paralysis resulting from brain injuries, theorized that fevers were often beneficial, correlated the wasting associated with syphilitic tabes with sexual activity, and provided the initial descriptions of human anthrax. Hippocrates advocated for the irrigation of wounds with wine and clean water, and insisted that physicians thoroughly clean their hands with hot water. He also emphasized the importance of working in well-lit settings, preferably with trained assistants, exclusively dedicated to surgical procedures.

These descriptions and treatments continued to be referred to well into the 17th century and are valuable as primary examples of observation and clinical diagnosis rather than experimental medicine works. Hippocrates, who had an unusually honest approach, considered the ability to predict an outcome as important as curing the patient, as evidenced by the fact that 60 percent of his 42 cases died.

Unlike the descriptive and surgical works, the theoretical portions of the Hippocratic corpus were based on errors and persisted for centuries. Illness and response to trauma were believed to be caused by an imbalance among the four humors: black bile, yellow bile, blood, and phlegm, which were associated with the four essential elements (earth, air, fire, and water). Treatments aimed at restoring balance, such as bleeding and purging, continued until the 19th century.

Hippocrates gained fame for his autonomy from religious faith and his reliance on observation. He advised physicians to consider various factors in regards to the patient, including their diet, occupation, and travel. He dismissed the notion that prayer, visions, miracles, or rituals had any impact on physical well-being. He outright rejected the idea that epilepsy was a "sacred disease." His emphasis on gathering information and making observations proved crucial for future researchers

Hippocrates, often referred to as the "Father of Medicine," observed and documented various medical conditions. In this case, he described inflammation, a biological response to injury or infection, with four characteristic signs:

1. Redness (rubor): This refers to an increased presence of blood in the affected area, leading to a reddish appearance. It is caused by the widening of blood vessels to allow immune cells and other substances to reach the site of injury or infection.
2. Heat (calor): Inflammation often generates warmth in the affected area. Increased blood flow as a result of vasodilation can lead to a sensation of heat.
3. Pain (dolor): Inflammation is typically accompanied by discomfort or pain at the site of injury or infection. This pain often arises due to the stimulation of nerve endings and the release of pain-inducing substances.
4. Swelling (tumor): Inflammation can lead to localized swelling or enlargement of the affected area. This occurs due to fluid accumulation and increased permeability of blood vessels, causing leakage of fluid and migration of immune cells.

Hippocrates' description of these four signs of inflammation provides a foundation for understanding this physiological response, and his observations have remained influential in medicine to this day. The understanding and identification of these characteristics continue to play a crucial role in diagnosing and managing inflammatory conditions.

Unlike Hippocrates, who was mainly an observer, Galen was a passionate dissector and experimenter. He dissected numerous animals, with a focus on apes for postmortem studies and pigs and dogs for live dissections. However, he applied himself to studying various species, including camels and elephants. Galen was one of the pioneers in experimenting on living organisms and he disproved Aristotle's belief that the brain only worked to cool the blood and that emotions resided in the heart.

Galen's experiments and discoveries were extensive and groundbreaking for his time. He performed different cuts on the spinal cord to produce various types of paralysis. In a live pig, he silenced its vocalization by severing the recurrent laryngeal nerve. Additionally, he demonstrated that a removed heart would continue to beat and a detached muscle would contract. Galen also proved that severing an optic nerve would result in blindness.

Galen served as a military surgeon alongside Marcus Aurelius and was able to distinguish between degenerative and traumatic aneurysms. He effectively controlled bleeding by locating the end of the severed vessel and either twisting or tying it on itself or suturing it with silk. Interestingly, this marked the first surgical use of silk, a rare material imported from the Orient that was primarily used for Roman women's wardrobes.

Combining his experimental findings with the philosophies of Hippocrates and Pythagoras, Galen developed an imaginative physiological system. However, as he only dissected animals and not humans, he made various anatomical errors that persisted in the medical literature for fifteen centuries following his death. Despite Galen's belief that students should always verify what they are taught, for the next 1,400 years, many individuals preferred to accept his writings without conducting their own observations or experiments.

We see that Hippocrates, who was mainly an observer, Galen was a passionate dissector and experimenter highlight that the same eastern medicine of an observer of natural cycle but from Galen is so different like modern western medicine concept

What is observer of eastern medicine by The HDNJ

HDNJ emphasizes treating the body as a whole and recognizes that each person has a unique pattern, requiring personalized treatment. Our bodies are not like cars, but rather resemble plants that follow the natural cycle. This distinction is a significant divergence in perspective. Western doctors fulfill a mechanic's role, while Eastern doctors resemble gardeners.

When it comes to building on yang, I would like to directly quote from the HDNJ. Yang Huang Di inquired, "The law of yin and yang is the natural order of the universe, the foundation and mother of all things, and the root of life and death. In healing, one must understand the root cause of disharmony, which is always influenced by the law of yin and yang." Qi Bo responded, "In the universe, pure yang qi rises to form heaven, while turbid yin Qi descends to create the earth. Yin is passive and quiet, while Yang is active and dynamic. Yang expands while Yin contracts, becoming astringent and solidifying. Yang represents energy, vital force, and potential, while yin represents substance, foundation, and the mother that gives birth to all potential."

Heaven generates Qi, while Earth gives rise to form. It is Heaven that regulates the four seasons. On Earth, the transformations of the five elements demonstrate the interaction of Yin and Yang. Yang ascends to create Heaven, while the murky Yin descends to shape the Earth. This movement contributes to the rhythm of the seasons and weather changes, allowing earthly things to manifest in the rhythm of birth in spring, growth in summer, consolidation in autumn, and storage in winter. With this knowledge, individuals can align their activities with these cycles and benefit from them, as human life is synchronized with its environment, Heaven, and Earth.

I think it is prescience philosophy that unseen area which modern western science did not recognize it means our body system is not fully defined by modern western science still working on with many side effects that happened so many unknown diagnoses.

The phenomenology of perceptions in eastern culture, as described in Nei jing, includes meteorology, phycology, astrology, the laws of the universe, the five elements theory, acupuncture, and moxibustion. These perspectives, which are from a long time ago, are still valid theories and philosophies that technology and biomedicine fail to acknowledge. Instead, they isolate cause and effect in laboratories, which goes against the teachings of Hagel.

another unique concept is the daoism

Daoism the way it is that follows the universal, cosmic principle like four seasons that we encounter every moment but how to do adapting situation

so it covers all symptoms to able to diagnosis by Cosmic Cycle

Contrary to many un diagnosis symptoms or syndrome that western medicine challenging these days

It is self contradictory of Western Medicine all symptom dissecting and isolating

Nai jing is more systematic with 8 differentiating symptoms that can diagnosis all of the diseases

Another the body of one who understands the dao will remain strong and healthy, the one who does not understand the dao will age

Those who understand the principles of wholesome living tame their minds and prevent them from straying. They do not force anything upon themselves or others, are happy and content tranquil and quiet, **can live indefinitely**. These are the ancient methods of self-maintenance"

I believe now is the perfect moment to revisit The HDNJ for the modern society more than ever before. As we navigate through the pandemic disaster, it is crucial to return to the fundamentals and examine the history of medicine to find a solution.

Modern society has deviated from fundamental natural approaches, often resorting to methods that involve dissecting and isolating the body, much like taking apart a car. However, we also recognize and celebrate the remarkable achievements that science has made across various fields. Western society often collaborates with Eastern philosophies, particularly in technology, leading to significant successes akin to those of major tech companies, except in the area of medicine.

Now is the time for Western medicine to embrace Eastern medicine and work together in harmony.

The lymphatic system starting and endpoint for viruses

I was impressed by the information "Enhancing lymphatic function for longevity" by Gerald M. Lenore. and Mark Hyman, MD's book, "Forever Young". Our lymphatic system is often overlooked in terms of our overall health. Despite being invisible and untouchable, it constantly works to eliminate metabolic waste from our tissues, which are the by-products of all our cellular processes.

Additionally, it plays a crucial role in absorbing fats from the gut and transporting them throughout our body, while also aiding in the movement of white blood cells to and from lymph nodes – crucial for fighting infections and cancer. Moreover, it serves as a link between our immune system and circulation by connecting lymph vessels to veins that lead to the heart. However, an imbalance in the lymphatic system can occur due to high consumption of processed foods, inadequate nutrient levels, and a lack of physical activity. It is important to emphasize that the lymph system is the beginning and end for viruses.

Without proper functioning of the lymphatic system, it is challenging to cure all virus diseases. However, the issue is often unseen and difficult to analyze in the lab using western medicine methods. Furthermore, vaccines are losing efficacy. So it is time to incorporated to eastern medicine and western medicine to figure unseen disease out why we have many information by eastern medicine to unseen factors

Harold clinic

Through the clinic all symptom root cause is malfunction of lymphatic system called lymphomas that have no medical help now

But I will provide many information to treatment option and why it matter to help them in detail

See it from western medicine view

lymphatic system, a subsystem of the circulatory systemin the vertebrate body that consists of a complex network of vessels, tissues, and organs. The lymphatic system helps maintain fluid balance in the body by collecting excess fluid and particulate matter from tissues and depositing them in the bloodstream

The essential function of lymph in the lungs is a fascinating topic for researchers. Recent studies have indicated that changes to the lymphatic system are present in almost all lung diseases. According to the article

"Lymphatics in Lung Disease," published by the National Institutes of Health in 2008, "The lymphatic circulation seems to play a crucial role in lung biology, both in health and in disease. ... Understanding the role of lymphatics in human lung disease is likely to enhance our understanding of disease pathogenesis and the development of therapeutic targets."

Throughout your body, lymph nodes are typically grouped around veins in adipose or other tissues. These nodes are where bacteria and viruses meet immune cells to mount a critical immune response. They may be as small as a pea or a kidney bean, but they are constantly surveilling your insides for any suspicious activity. Healthy lymph nodes can vary in size from 2 millimeters to 2.5 centimeters in diameter. Since lymph nodes do not regenerate, surgical removal, typically due to cancer treatment, can lead to mechanical insufficiency, impairing the body's ability to eliminate excess lymphatic fluid. This can increase the risk of developing lymphedema and other lymphatic system disorders.

In the treatment plan I emphasized Lymph nodes within the lungs and the mediastinum location where most primary infection occur for breathing issue. So always check the sternum in chest with finger some uncomfortable or pain need attention for sure

I will explain more in detail next chapter

Lymphatic fluid is brought into the lymph nodes through afferent lymphatic vessels. Macrophages within the nodes work to filter out bacteria.

Lymph nodes within the lungs and the mediastinum, the membranous partition between the lungs, perform their filtering function before the lymph is returned to the blood through bronchomediastinal trunks.

We need more information for lymphatic system cause it is basic fundamental information that we have to know

As a fetus develops, stem cells that will become white blood cells and lymphocytes are formed in the bone marrow and migrate to lymphoid organs throughout your body--which you probably didn't realize are part of the lymphatic system

These lymphoid organs--your bone marrow, tonsils and adenoids, thymus, **mucosa-associated lymphoid tissue (MALT)**, gut associated lymphoid tissue (GALT), spleen, appendix, Peyer's patches, and urinary tract--are small masses of lymph tissue found where a Mucous Membranes of Respiratory lot of bacteria tends to accumulate, so they are close by in order

As you see There are many lymphoid organs that we have as a clinic point of view the root cause of lymphoma starting in

GALT (gut associated lymphoid, Lymphoid Tissue) that first safeguards of your immune system

Again, Fifty percent of lymphoid tissue falls under the umbrella term mucosa-associated lymphoid tissue (MALT), including the digestive, urinary, and respiratory tracts: it filters debris that is passed through your skin or the mucous.

Over all I am clear that the digestive lymphoid tissue is the root cause of all virus disease through the clinic

What is functional medicine?

It emphasizes unity and wholeness.emphasizes unity and wholeness

Western medicine incorporates concepts similar to functional medicine found in eastern medicine.

Functional medicine is the ability to perceive the situation of its activities without a physical form.

Functional problems like migraine, fatigue, mental illness, colitis, rheumatism, asthma, and menstrual cramps are often considered psychosomatic. This means that they cannot be proven to originate in the body and are believed to be influenced by psychological factors. This perspective suggests that the root cause and manifestation of these issues are not solely physical but also involve psychological aspects that impact overall well-being.

The intricate relationship between the mind and body plays a crucial role in leading to these conditions. This suggests that understanding and addressing underlying psychological factors, such as stress, emotions, and beliefs, may be necessary for managing or resolving these issues.

Functional medicine focuses on asking two main questions to identify the root cause of dysfunction in the body's ecosystem and determining what is needed to restore balance. Essentially, it aims to comprehend how the body's exposome either hinders or promotes its overall health.

I will provide an example of a functional medicine case focusing on the lung from both perspectives.

In the book "Breath Taking" by Michael J. Stepen, Dr. Avery was studying bubbles and surface tension of lung tissue. while a group of dedicated scientists, employed by the federal government during the Cold War, were researching the lung's response to chemical warfare. Since the lungs are a common entry point for poisonous gases, comprehending how toxins impact the lungs and how to combat them was a priority. Dr. John Clements, a researcher at the Army base in Bethesda, Maryland, conducted experiments in the mid-1950s to quantitatively measure lung tissue's surface tension. His experiments revealed that lung tissue had significantly lower surface tension compared to other tissues. Furthermore, he conducted a groundbreaking experiment by measuring pressure changes in extracted lung tissue during expansion and contraction, a feat never before accomplished.

As mentioned, the pressure on a sphere like a soap bubble or a lung alveolus is proportional to its surface tension divided by its radius, and lower pressures will mean the bubble will have a greater chance of not collapsing in on itself. Remarkably, the pressure decreased significantly with lung contraction as the alveoli in the lung were getting smaller. The blood then travels into the right side of our heart, which pumps it to our lungs. From there, it travels to the left side of the heart to be pumped through the rest of the body.

However, if the left chamber of the heart fails, as often happens with cardiac disease, the blood backs up into the lungs and fluid spills out into the alveoli. Laennec noticed that in a certain subset of people, fluid was spilling into the lungs without heart failure or high pressure. The capillaries of the lung were simply leaky, and patients were essentially drowning.

When comparing the surface tension of the lungs from a Western perspective, Eastern medicine offers a broader perspective by considering the triple burner meridian in the whole body for tension. Let's examine what the triple bunner meridian looks like first. Why is it called triple? Why the number 3? The number three symbolizes completion in Eastern medicine, Born from the growth and completion of one cycle, the three-dimensional, triangle and The Holy Trinitythe even an atom in Western medicine consists of protons, neutrons, and electrons. I will elaborate further on this theory in subsequent chapters.

Now, let's go back to the Triple Burner meridian. We refer to it as the upper respiratory system because the upper, middle, and lower systems exist and are combined to make it whole.The first upper respiratory system includes the lungs and heart working together to distribute oxygen from the atmosphere throughout the body in an invisible cycle called the fog cycle. An acupuncture point associated with this system is Danjung located at the center of the sternum between the nipples

The second part of the Triple Burner meridian is the middle digestion system, which includes the stomach and spleen. These organs absorb food from the diaphragm to the navel, with an invisible energy function similar to mist.

The third part is the source system, known as the lower Jiao. This system extends from the belly to the anus and includes the liver, kidney, small intestine, and large intestine. The essence of the body's water, called Jing, is an essential aspect of this system.

Clinic Case of functional case

I had a patient his name Richard in his 50th
> He looks healthy with good food looks like no issue by outside no scar
> but he complains pain in the neck seems like he cannot pull back smoothly
> so are okay put the acupuncture needle in the pain location I ask because he feel afraid of acupuncture treatment

he agrees and just one needle insert the location and just waiting 10 minutes

after taking it out how do you feel he looks like a little surprised neck pain gone

his neck structure is strong, but his functioning of neck is not

as build up trust

he tells me all medical history

he complains nose congestion frequently in the morning waking up sleep and next neck and shoulder pain

left kidney stone in 2018 right heart arrythmia in 2014

the catching my eye is sensitive bowl movement digestion issue and gout

as I mention in the lymphatic system it seems that the root cause of all system is the sensitive bowl movement

why I mention early the gut in small intestine that produce the main lymph fluids is infected invisibly

I think the rest of all symptom is derived from gut make it simple you need to take care of bowl with fresh detox fruits first like apple ginger garlic onion for invisible attacking your gut some detox supplement out there

Make it simple the first is your gut no doubt the rest is healing itself accordingly

The Meridian is the blueprint for the body's electrical lines

This system is unique and crucial for the treatment of all diseases, even though it is not well-known in Western medicine. The importance of Meridian Theory lies in its ability to make all symptoms treatable and aid in diagnosis, much like referring to a manual book for a washing machine or checking the electrical box for a power outage.

According to Meridian Theory in Traditional Chinese Medicine (TCM), the system of channels or pathways through which Qi flows is essential. These specific meridians connect the organs and various parts of the body, creating a network that allows for the communication and regulation of organ energy.

There are six Yang and six Yin meridians in the body. The functions of these channels are considered to be like antennas that receive cosmic influence and transmit it into the body. The flow of Qi in the channels always moves from distal (coming from the exterior, entering at the tips of the extremities like the fingers for qi and toes for blood Yin) to proximal (towards the center, flowing towards the internal organs).

The main channels mirror the 12 earthly branches and the 10 heavenly branches. I will delve more deeply into this topic in the next book, as it is complex and requires more time to fully explain.

Each primary channel, along with its corresponding secondary channels, creates a complex and multi-layered organizational unit known as a "meridian system". These systems establish various relationships and connections.

However, when people receive acupuncture stimulation, they feel sensations that move along the same routes as the meridians. This was called '순경감전 (Meridian Conduction Sensation)'. In the 1970s, people conducted in-depth research on meridian conduction sensation and discovered peculiar characteristics such as "it is slow, at a few centimeters per second; the sensation of meridian conduction is blocked when mechanically pressured or injected with saline; it is directed towards areas with distinct disease symptoms." It wasn't until the 1980s that objective proof through CT imaging was achieved. It was discovered that there are physical properties in the meridian lines that allow for electrical resistance, vibration, heat conduction, and isotope transition.

For example Cough into your arm and feel the coldness in your arm's long sleeve. Why wear a turtleneck? Where three fung (wind) sensor points? Why feel cold in the arm? It's the air sensor. Designed by meridian or something else, we gather a lot of information about meridian.

It is also called the Twelve Regular Meridians (十二正經) compared to the Eight Extraordinary Vessels (奇經八脈). The 12 regular meridians and the 8 extraordinary vessels generally flow in a vertical upward and downward direction in the body. Distribution, hand (手), foot (足).

Fingers play a crucial role as they serve as the primary connection to celestial energy, akin to the branches of a tree. Utilizing our hands and fingers positively stimulates the brain and can even slow down the aging process, as it is inherently linked to our breathing—a fundamental vital function. Regular finger exercises, such as push-ups with your fingers or gripping movements, can significantly enhance strength and dexterity.

Consider the practice of playing the piano; it exemplifies why hand coordination is beneficial. When we stretch our fingers, we promote circulation and flexibility, which are essential after a night's sleep. Stretching our fingers and hands in bed can prepare our bodies for the day ahead, enhancing our breathing and overall vitality.

Every morning, inhaling fresh oxygen and stretching his entire body inspires you to generate new ideas and embrace the day ahead.

considering it from a Western perspective., various types of nerves, including the vagus nerve, as well as the parasympathetic and sympathetic nerves, are intricately interconnected. Additionally, cranial nerves play a part in this complex network. Because of these interconnections, it is often challenging to distinguish between nerves and blood vessels, contributing to a sense of overall wholeness in the body's systems

The Bluenose Marathon

The Bluenose Marathon takes place in Halifax, a small town peninsula surrounded by ocean basins, making it quiet with a combination of the Public Garden In 1850 and new great buildings. It is a big tradition of known as a Haligonian.

Early in the morning in 2018, the race starts downtown, passing through Point Pleasant Mountain, South and North, neighboring towns all around Halifax. All the residents cheer on by saying "Go Harold, go Harold".

Going uphill at a 50-degree angle at Point Pleasant Park is challenging, but okay. Following big music cheers by volunteers, snatching a couple of energy bars helps to feel good again.

After completing one round, pain in my groin area bothers me. In the last couple of years during this race, I was fine, went home, and slept like a dog to recover. But this time, the pain doesn't go away, so I stop, walk, stop, walk, and end up with a problem because I didn't take proper care of it. That was my mistake.

according to the book : The wisdom of body by Walter Bradford Cannon

This book is great to use the terms of oxygen debt in 1930 very scientific terms with economical language

When he engages in intense muscular effort, the amount of oxygen intake may rise to 15 liters per minute or even higher. However, even under the most favorable circumstances, the maximum amount of oxygen that can be taken in and utilized by the body is only 4 liters per minute.

Therefore, during vigorous exercise, the intake of oxygen can be 10 to 12 times greater than at rest and still fall short of what is actually needed at that time.

the lactic acid that is produced during muscle contractions cannot be converted into carbon dioxide or transformed back into its precursor, glycogen. As a result, it accumulates in the muscles. Although muscular contractions can still occur, their efficiency decreases due to the higher concentration of lactic acid, which interferes with the contractile process. This indicates that intense exertion does not rely solely on immediate oxidation.

For example, the lactic acid we generate during intense efforts, like a 225 yards run, is temporarily neutralized in the muscles and fluid matrix. Only later is it burned or transformed back into its precursor form.

But almost all of it is burned or reconverted into glycogen. This burning occurs after the exercise has ceased. We therefore borrow the ability to go on working beyond the limit set by the oxygen available, but only on condition that we take in enough oxygen later to burn the accumulated waste. We thus run up what Hill has called an "oxygen debt." We pay the debt during the continued deep respiration

Energy debt in the body

Two-thirds of all energy expended actually goes towards sustaining life. This is known as the basic metabolic rate (BMR). It always surprises me how much energy this requires. Having enough energy for BMR poses a particular challenge for people because they lack sufficient energy for basic metabolism. As a result, they may experience mild multiple organ failure simply due to an energy deficiency. Essential organs, such as the kidneys, are relatively protected. The clinical assumption is that when energy expenditure exceeds delivery, entering negative territory, organs may begin to fail and symptoms may appear.

With two-thirds of our energy dedicated to BMR, one-third is left for physical, mental, and essential evolutionary functions.

Understanding the concept of energy debt and its impact using economic terms

Energy is valuable, like money - it is hard-earned and enjoyable to spend. However, we can run into serious financial (or rather, energy) problems when our demand exceeds our delivery. In this case, we can borrow energy using beneficial techniques. However, this comes at a cost.

First, we experience the pain of lactic acid buildup, and second, we accumulate an energy debt that needs to be repaid with interest - to be precise, the interest rate is 300 percent.

This is similar to borrowing energy (or money) from a loan shark in life - all our energy (or money) is used to catch up (paying the interest), leaving us with not enough for recovery.

Pacing is essential to maintain a positive energy balance. If we do not pace ourselves properly and fall into an energy deficit, we can.

In conclusion, it is best not to be either a borrower or a lender in the realm of energy.

What happens when energy demand exceeds energy delivery?

The most efficient way to produce energy is by burning the fuel acetate in mitochondria with oxygen. Acetate is ideally derived from ketones, but glucose can also be used. This process is known as aerobic metabolism and is highly efficient. One molecule of acetate generates 32-36 molecules of ATP, our universal energy currency, depending on the system's efficiency.

The statement "Acetate is ideally derived from ketones, but glucose can also be used" refers to the metabolic processes in the body where acetate, a type of molecule, can be obtained either from the breakdown of ketones or from glucose metabolism.

Overall, the statement highlights the flexibility of the body's metabolic processes, noting that acetate can be obtained from both ketones and glucose, depending on the body's metabolic state, energy requirements, and nutrient availability.

If energy demand surpasses delivery, there are at least two alternative ways to produce ATP, but they are both extremely inefficient, as previously mentioned. It can take hours, or even days, for normal aerobic metabolism to be restored. This catch-up process involves painful lactic acid buildup and a significant increase in energy demands because one must not only repay the debt but also deal with additional crippling interest rates.

For those who have the time, energy, and interest in biochemistry, the detailed biochemical explanation will follow.

These two types of energy are produced in different muscle fibers throughout the body. As anaerobic respiration is intended as a backup system, our bodies have fewer anaerobic muscle fibers. Relying too heavily on these less-developed muscles can eventually lead to breakdown and injury.

Anaerobic energy is produced solely through the use of glucose, a simple sugar. It is a quicker and easier process for our bodies to access, serving as a backup system and providing a boost when oxygen is lacking.

However, anaerobic energy is inefficient and can lead to the production of excess lactic acid. The discomfort experienced after pushing oneself too hard at the gym, such as nausea, muscle weakness, and sweating, is the result of anaerobic overload.

This is why the initial minutes of an intense workout are often unpleasant - our lungs and respiratory system have not caught up to supply the necessary oxygen, so the body must rely on anaerobic respiration. As we warm up and progress in our exercise, the body switches to aerobic respiration, explaining why it becomes easier.

In my experience with runner's pain, I've come to understand that many people often push themselves to exercise beyond their limits. This approach is misguided, especially when you're not getting enough oxygen. If you experience pain, it's important to stop immediately. Just because you feel okay temporarily doesn't mean the issue has resolved. In my case, the pain recurs, and I realize it is quite serious.

Explore a deeper understanding of groin pain from a Western perspective, as marathon runners are well aware of its implications.

let's consider the anatomy related to the lymphatic system and the femoral nerve. The femoral nerve innervates the anterior compartment of the thigh. The femoral sheath comprises the femoral artery and its branches, which supply blood to the majority of the lower limb, as well as the femoral vein, into which the great saphenous vein drains within the femoral triangle. The femoral canal contains lymph nodes and vessels.

Regarding inguinal hernias, they typically occur when fatty tissue or a segment of the bowel, such as the intestine, protrudes through a weak spot in the abdominal wall into the groin, specifically through an area known as the inguinal canal. These hernias predominantly affect men. An inguinal hernia that cannot be repositioned back into the abdomen is termed an incarcerated hernia, which presents a serious health risk

From the eastern medicine point of view
It is the stagnation of Liver-Qi arises toxic build up through the excess over do running beyond your limit by breathing oxygen deficiency and clogging blood circulation
Both groin area is the meridian of liver channel to detox function of inner body cleansing so pain express something wrong
Running science of eastern medicine just the liver and gallbladder organ involving muscle and ligament,muscle feeding by blood
simple put it without blood it cramp like no oil in the car
Gallbladder meridian is the main lateral both including sciatic nerve all muscle and ligament is placed lateral side of both leg fundamental of running
The Gallbladder meridian similarly to a running muscle, with soft contractions and releases that are essential for the smooth transformation

needed in running. It is interesting to note why the term "bluenose" is used instead of "white nose" or "black nose". In Eastern medicine, the color blue represents the liver and gallbladder organs, symbolizing the start of something. Blue also has connections to the east.

The Bluenose schooner, a 50-meter long boat in Lunenburg, Nova Scotia, holds the same meaning as it did in the 19th century. The Bluenose marathon starts on Sackville Road, named after the WW2 war ship that boarded 123 people to fight enemy U-boats during the war

Three defense systems from Eastern and Western Medicine

In the Western viewpoint, the three types of cells involved in phagocytosis are macrophages, neutrophils, and dendritic cells. When the body is invaded by a pathogen, an immune response is triggered by antigens, leading to the production of specific antibodies. Mast cells, macrophages, and neutrophils play roles in inflammation within the immune system.

The spleen, which filters blood as opposed to lymph like lymph nodes, has a structure similar to lymph nodes. The first line of defense against pathogens includes the skin, lysozyme, and normal microbiota.

First Line of Defense: Skin, Lysozyme, Normal Microbiota
Second Line of Defense: Neutrophils, Inflammation
Third Line of Defense: Plasma/B Cells, Antibodies, T Helper Cells

Lymph does not come directly from fluid leaked out of blood vessels. It is derived from interstitial fluid that is collected by lymphatic vessels in tissues.

Interstitial fluid refers to the fluid found in the interstitial spaces, which are the spaces between the cells and tissues of the body. It fills the gaps between cells and surrounds them, acting as a medium for the exchange of nutrients, waste products, and gases.

The interstitial fluid is derived from the blood plasma. It is a clear, watery fluid that contains various substances such as ions, nutrients, gases, hormones, and waste products. It serves as a transport medium, allowing for the exchange of these substances between the blood and the cells.

The movement of substances between the blood and the interstitial fluid is facilitated by small blood vessels called capillaries, which have permeable walls that allow for the exchange of molecules. Oxygen, nutrients, and other essential substances are transported from the capillaries into the interstitial fluid to nourish the cells, while waste products and carbon dioxide are eliminated in the reverse direction.

Overall, interstitial fluid plays a crucial role in maintaining the balance and health of cells by providing them with necessary nutrients and removing waste products. It serves as the intermediary between the blood and the cells, facilitating the exchange of essential substances for cellular function.

Lymph is not directly derived from fluid leaked out of blood vessels. It is actually collected from interstitial fluid by lymphatic vessels in tissues. Cells are important components of our internal immune system, but other factors such as antibodies, cytokines, and complement proteins also play crucial roles. Antigen-presenting cells (APCs), such as dendritic cells, macrophages, and B cells, do not directly interact with mast cells.

The first line of defense is located on the exterior of our body, known as the Taeyang cold symptom foot bladder meridian where one may feel cold and excrete more urine. The hand small intestine meridian may show lower bowel pain. The heavenly sensor of the body for defense is Du-16 Fengfu just below the base of the skull at the nape area where the neck meets the head.Wind Palace, which is a Nature Point of the Yang Linking Vessel (Yang Wei Mai). This point functions to extinguish interior Wind, and benefit the Brain, calm the Mind and open the Mind's orifices.

The second defense line is found between the exterior and interior, known as the soyang cold symptom foot gallbladder meridian which may exhibit muscle pain, cold and heat alternating symptoms, and feelings of low energy. The hand triple burner meridian includes BL-12 Fengmen Wind Door. BL-12 Fengmen is in line with the lower border of the spinous process of the first thoracic vertebra

The third defense line is located in the interior and is the deepest level of defense against pathogens.

The condition is known as Yangmyung cold symptoms, affecting the foot small intestine meridian and hand large intestine meridian. It is characterized by blood level symptoms like high heat, vomiting, brain fog, and bad mouth smell. The hand large intestine meridian displays cold lower bowel, diarrhea, and urinary incontinence.

Why does the triple burner and large intestine affect deeper levels? The G.B.-20 Fengchi Wind Pool located at the base of the skull, in the hollow just behind each ear. expel exterior Wind, extinguish interior Wind, subdue Liver-Yang, brighten the eyes, benefit the ears, and clear Heat.

To sum up The first pathogen entered the body through the spinal cord, known as the Bladder meridian, and passed through the skin on the back. It then traveled to the muscle meridian, causing muscle pain. Eventually, it reached the blood and viscera levels, leading to more severe symptoms like vomiting.

The Harold Clinic

I believes in the unique Meridian theory, which provides valuable information for self-treatment. It offers a different perspective compared to Western medicine, focusing on cellular level

In clinical trials, acupuncture points can provide useful information. Why do people wear turtleneck sweaters? Why do they experience finger and toe pain during covid symptom? The first symptom is typically a dislike for cold temperatures, which is common among patients.

When these three points are working well, we are interconnected to heavenly energy, which is good for basic health and oxygen. However, if these points are not functioning properly, it can lead to coughing, colds, and runny noses instantly. It is important to always check these points and practice skin breathing or forest bathing for optimal health.

Five Organs (Zang) and Six Fu Organs (Fu)

Five Organs (Zang) are considered solid organs responsible for storing and maintaining bodily functions called yin organ

Six Fu Organs (Fu) are hollow organs that facilitate the transport and excretion called yang organ
the five viscera and six bowels

again, western medicine focus Cell tissue and eastern medicine starting organ base

The twelve main meridians are located inside the arms, with lungs, heart, and pericardium meridians located inside the forearm, and large intestine, small intestine, and triple burner meridians located outside the forearm, extending as six meridians.

On the inside of the foot are kidney, bladder, liver, and stomach meridians, with bladder and gallbladder meridians located on the back of the foot, making a total of 12 meridians that correspond to the five viscera and six bowels,

The thoracic bone, also known as the back bone, is critical for the upper three bones which encompass the heart and lungs. The sympathetic nerve goes to the yang side,

The interaction between the heart and lungs is known to be controlled by the autonomous nervous system, which is responsible for controlling the cervical 4, 5, 6, 7, nasal tonsils, pharynx, trachea, asthma, and thyroid glands. It is also responsible for controlling the innervation of the upper limbs as the main nerves of the heart are connected to the upper limb nerves.

The liquid nerves and muscular nerves, including vasomotor nerves, radicular nerves, and spinal nerves, control all the nerves related to the hand. This can be seen when the heart nerve of the fifth finger, lung nerve of the thumb, and large intestine nerve of the index finger work together.

Therefore, the sudden tingling in the fingers after a meal has a similar effect of increasing oxygen supply.

Wind and Unwind

Wind is the breath of nature, embodying an energy that is taken seriously in Eastern medicine. It is not simply referred to as "wind"; rather, it is categorized into six types: cold wind, warm wind, damp wind, dry wind, and cold wind. We sense these six types of wind through three key acupuncture points: Fungmun, Fungji, and Fungfu.

Wind is stage 3 damaging pathogens condition that shaking limb and severe disease with stroke win damp cold like tornado ripping up roof blow away all things even kill m the people so tremble by stroke toxic inside wind win damp cold like toxic mucus so on so bad meaning in eastern medicine so western unwind relax like meditation opposite so right

Eastern medicine says

this clinical characteristic of Wind is Sudden rigidity is due to Wind." This refers to the clinical manifestations resulting from both interior and exterior.

Wind affects the skin, cause a large number of skin diseases characterized by generalized itching, affliction of the top of the body, skin rashes with sudden onset and development. (i.e. eczema; pruritus; stroke; epilepsy)

So External Wind affects the Lungs first and internal Wind affects the Liver

Wind is Yang in nature and tends to injure Blood and Yin.

Wind is often the vehicle through which other climatic factors invade the body.

For example: Cold will often enter the body as Wind-Cold and Heat as Wind-Heat. The clinical manifestation of Wind mimic the action of wind itself in Nature: the Wind arises quickly and changes rapidly. It moves swifly, blows intermittently and sways the top of trees.

Wind causes invonluntary movements in the form of tremors or convulsions

Wind can also cause the opposite: paralysis and rigidity

First, the most crucial point is the name of the Wind

Also western book "Between Heaven and Earth" by Ted Kaptchuk describes the wind

"Wind characterized by aversion to drafts, sudden change, spasms, disequilibrium, tears, migratory pains, dizziness, trembling, stuffy nose, scratchy, throat, and numbness

Another Book "Decoding Ba-gua and I – Ching Origin Enigma" by Antoine Khai Nguyen

Wind Deity based on the sun and Moon to produce divinatory texts appeared in the same time with the creation of primitive Chinese character

Western medicine wind

Air is the incorporeal, abstract element. Therefore, it has many complex associations and meanings. In terms of the substances we breathe, air has a specific composition. It is made up of 78% nitrogen, 21% oxygen, and trace amounts of carbon dioxide, water vapor, and inert gases. Additionally, air can also refer to the atmosphere that surrounds the Earth. It can represent both breath and wind, which is often considered as nature's breath. When people express their opinions publicly, they are said to voice their thoughts "in the air," giving air connotations of expression and revelation.

Furthermore, air can also be used to describe various artistic forms, such as music, dance, or writing, adding a lively and colorful aspect to this word.

When something is described as being "in the air" or "up in the air," it means that it is uncertain or not yet fixed. This not only creates a sense of ambiguity but also generates anticipation. Individuals who are said to "walk on air" are often extremely happy. While having an air of confidence can be seen as complimentary, pretending to have an air of superiority is negative and filled with empty promises. The word "airy" can describe someone or something that is light, breezy, and lofty, but it can also suggest a flaky and highly speculative nature, similar to "building castles in the air."

As one of the four elemental forces, air's nature contributes to many fundamental associations. Although air is stable in its purest form, its composition can change with increasing altitude and in enclosed spaces used by plants and animals. Air is undoubtedly essential for life on Earth, blending harmoniously with other elements.

Harold clinic

Wind air is the environment of cosmic energy meaning each air wind had their own invisible energy that affecting your body condition so healthy person well adjusting external energy some are not catch a cold runny nose

All functional medicine take accounting all invisible factor like virus air wind and lymphatic system that is matter nowadays

We can only just feel it. All deferent feeling by each person so we accept that all depends on each personal body condition

Heart Lung transformation principle
The first basic theory of eastern medicine

It is unique theory of eastern medicine explain body structure by natural order

To comprehensively comprehend this transformation and its reasons, as explained by Evans, we must journey back in time, well before Homo sapiens even existed.

Make it simple

Like the vehicle motor engine and fan relationship to cooling off the car heat fan is located covering the engine in front bonnet

excess heat of engine broken down the car some cold winter we pre heating the engine to heat up

The same principle of human

See the location of lung and heart it meant to be Left lung 2 lobes and right lung 3 why is that mean because of heart

So left side of body represented heart call the blood

right side of body call the breathing or qi or invisible energy find out checking wrist pulse of basic diagnosis

again

So left wrist pulse shows the blood condition

Right wrist pulse is shows qi or breathing condition it is basic diagnosis of eastern medicine meaning the pulse is strong the blood and energy condition is good it not blood or energy is sluggish the same feeling of pulse that is simple and easy diagnosis a little in detail left wrist show the three part liver heart and kidney yin right wrist three part shows the lung kidney yang

Eastern medicine by 5 elementary theory lung is metal heart is fire element so located in the most active area due to its role in the exchange of metal and fire, it forms the functions of the heart and lung, maintaining balance between fire and breathing oxygen. Again It forms the functions of the heart and lung, by converging the actions of breathing air and regulating the heat of fire.

The lungs correspond to the Yin of the great meridian and represent autumn. They are dry and have white skin and fur with a white nasal cavity.

The interaction between the heart and the lungs is known to be controlled by the autonomic nerves responsible for the cervical vertebrae 4, 5, 6, and 7, the nasal tonsils, the pharyngeal tonsils, the bronchi, asthma, sea coral, thyroid gland, and adrenal medulla.

Therefore, the correlation and interaction between the heart and lungs are the most crucial factors in respiration.

I share 3 case of clinic with heart and lung relationship disease that is important for basic covid and chronic disease

Clinic case 1

Heart heat > lung contraction

Her name is jane in her 30th from rural area in nova scotia who is single mom with 2 kids living with her mom together

Chief complaint: Hard to breathing

Medical history: she has a chronic respiratory symptom getting worse from 7 years ago hard to breathing with energy burning out and uncontrollable emotion

Surgery : Left leg surgery last year that is planned to

She got treatment for local TCM practitioner treatment for chronic symptom for 7 years

Exercise and movement : She try to take a walk in the morning

Eating and drinking : Eating fruits drinking a lot every day for nourishing the Yin against the internal heat She feels hungry most of time and it digests quickly after eating

Her herbal formula by Herbalist that is intreating to me cause a little different from what TCM's herb concoction
I like to share real information any clinic case and it is true story so I give you a detail information

Here is the formular :
Rosemary. Blood circulation for inflammatory Licorice : Reducing body fat, healing ulcer
Lobelia : For respiratory with blue color affecting low blood Cinnamon : Losing belly fat
Artic root : Loss weight Vervain : For insomnia and depression with pink color
Chaste tree. : Blooming on late summer for menstrual cycle, Stimulates

Objective finding: She is so unique constitution tendency
Her hand feels cold that seems like fake cold because her pulse is so strong at right arm and a little different in left arm
heart and liver position of pulse feels so strong and Kidney Yin position feels empty
It means Yin Deficiency by excess heat drying up the body fluids that she drinks frequently and more bad to lung
Heart fire attacking the Lung causing breathing issue, hard to breath.
Fire elements making her mood like kinds of all or nothing pattern,3 days hyper vibe and 3 days collapsing feeling on and on
Sleep : Half week is okay but the other week is not good sleeping quality

She likes to get together with two kids and her mother to talk

Clinic

Very interesting thing in the clinic at 5th time

When acupuncture in the skull and face I feel it her inside heat radiating so unique constitution that her hand feels cold that seems like fake cold.

meaning I do the right diagnosis, and she agree that heat up and down affecting her condition

I told her you need harmonizing and balancing so drastically because you born in significant Yang Excess

She feels that it affected positive respond for her breathing and menstrual cycle

I comment that some ingredient is negative impact that drying up your body fluids

So, she like to feedback to herbalist

Interesting thing is some herb come from England .why England Eastern boutique is so popular I will explain in chapter 3

First thing to this patient, taking fresh fruit whatever you want to go grocery and try it all kinds of fruits first

Make it simple you are in fire always so bring the water to cool off. Nourish low level of body fluids and eat fish go jumping ocean and forest breathing

Stay in nature as much as you can to calm the flaring heat

This case is unique in terms of breathing case meaning is not the chronic and covid case

Heart, lung balancing case

Clinic Case 2

His name is john in his 50th a little heart heat than lung yin balance meaning his heat and lung well balance

How to know that see the 5 elementary theory in chapter to know the 5 organ energy allocation by your birth day

He like Sports early age and good body shape

He go to the gym fitness 4 early morning with blueberry cocktail drinking

He do not like heat on summer go fishing hate to mosquito that love his blood heat

he is okay for western treatment like surgery and taking pill when he is sick visiting family doctor get prescription

he get all vaccine and flu shot as well

he work at manager of big distribution company very good memory remembering 300 items price each year

in terms of his breathing way more exhale power so he like to talk continue to talk meaning lung breathing function well

he can read other buyer mind through the eye and good business negotiator

he is blood type o

He is still energetic and making love with girlfriend

This is the case of heart and lung balance type of person

and his girlfriend had no vaccine at all during the pandemic she is real vegetarian based on the religion interesting thing is she is very good immune condition no room to covid virus settle in

she is a little tired after work cause not enough of protein, but her immune system is above than normal and not much toxic inside in her age

it is from her good diet pattern and circulation well for lymph system function well

She is strict to her diet eventually very good condition in her 50th

Very clear that what do you eat meaning what your gut condition is all about no matter what kind of virus invade

Defense system first and taking calorie second

The last case is particularly vulnerable to the most recent strain of COVID-19.

Heart heat < lung contraction

this is the case of virus disease case

Make it simple not enough body heat meaning ATP function below than normal why it is gene

This book is for this type of patients

put another word lung is excess reduce the body heat and contracting your blood vessel causing blood circulation issue

this case is vulnerable to the virus of cold pattern

Meaning all lower body heat lower ATP causing digestion issue and easy to acidic to free radical

This case is more option eastern medicine to treat why more side effect of medication and surgery because liver function detox is lower than normal

What is other option

Make it simple the first thing to treat is heat up body on purpose so Japan tiny moxibustion and hot therapy and infrared heat sauna or hot tub all kinds of heat infusion to your skin See the skin 3rd brain and gut digestion 2nd brain next chapter

Case

Both case adam 2 type of person see the gene and environment

She is her 30th

She got surgery back alongside left upper to middle gastrointestinal that causing the dampness more serious

She did not treat properly so she feel pain that surgery stitch line.

It got worse when it cold or rainy day

Another fact is that she used to late night eating causing dampness

She frequently feels hungry and eating more than normal with emotional fact

Blood circulation issue metabolism ATP function below the normal so less oxygen intake with nutrition

Mostly this type is all circulation issue

She is not getting the answer from western medicine

Spleen and St heat deficiency with Dampness

It looks like Sp Xu St Yang Def with def of Heart heat Xu prevent her from proper nutrition metabolism

Surgery is bad to her it affecting whole your life still many toxic is in her inside

She is still young and good time to detox

But when you get older more your immune system decline more time to heal

She is lung excess type vulnerable to the virus

Treatment plan

Increasing SP Qi and Yang.

Tonifying Heart blood and fire body heat

Increasing Body heat for blood circulation to resolve the Dampness

Ren 5, 6 Japanese tiny Moxa

Back Shu point for dealing with Yang Qi to tonified the middle Jaio

Tonify the St and Sp Qi with Moxa St 36

Damp stagnation Sp 6

Second case

Jenny is her mid 30th single mom with 6 years daughter so cute active and running here there

She is chronic pain in the shoulder and all negative emotion capture her feel depression

in the first clinic she need some help to combat lose hair and insomnias so on

Simply put it she malfunctions of the liver detox inside and not enough of oxygen breathing so it accumulates

See the oxygen breathing chapter 2

she try to find answer in eastern medicine why western do not give her any answer

So she is in acupuncture course to learn more hope find the answer

Regarding Insomnia see the rem sleep chapter

Her type is susceptible to viruses when there is a lack of smooth flow, leading to imbalances or blockages. Stagnation—whether physical, emotional, or spiritual—can eventually manifest as disease. Picture yourself as a jellyfish, drawing in qi and releasing it.

She advocates for what she calls "health and wellness snacking," which refers to one- or two-minute practices such as body tapping or "rescue breathing," where you take deep, meditative breaths to alleviate stress.

In this way, Traditional Chinese Medicine (TCM) can seamlessly integrate into your life, becoming a natural part of your routine. Health is not found in a potion, powder, or pill; it is comprised of the small daily actions that accumulate over time.

She is quiet and shy and easy to catch a cold

She is some signal in the lymph system issue

Mainly some stress affected her Liver Qi and blood it affected all body system negatively

First, Shoulder stiffness is serious GB 21 and both side of neck muscle is tightness

First acupuncture treatment she feels relived the GB 21 pain instantly

I perceive needle feeling in GB 21 not like jelly smooth muscle when I insert the needle

Following manipulating technic to attack the muscle spasm by three or four-times quick vibration vertically

I think it worked out and she agreed on that

Next job is in the neck spasm both side that is related to shoulder pain

Generally, neck muscle stiffness and shoulder pain goes together

She is interested in reiki practice

She is smart and good writer but more negative prone to because heart heat energy is not enough comparing the lung

So feeling negative dragging down by excess lung compered to liver moving up energy

Harold clinic

Eastern medicine make it simple

the qi or oxygen breathing flows and the blood moves meaning yang energy flows and yin blood moves

Circulation needs to move smoothly round your body, just as much for your qi as for your blood. To promote this, shake your arms, legs, and whole body for a minute. You can also tap all over your body whenever you feel sluggish, using a slightly clenched fist or bamboo wand, to stimulate and invigorate your cells and unblock your qi.so check first oxygen breathing second wrist pulse

the brachial plexus and the lung medidian

lung meridian starting first in circadin rhythum

why the lung medidian is so imprtotant because of breathing

interesting thing is that starting point of lung meridian is the lymph node below the clavicle so great related to the lymphstic system

western view called the braichal plexus

The eastern perspective of the lung meridian is characterized by its yin nature. It ascends from the brachial plexus to the thumb and descends from the index finger, aligning with the large intestine channel. A particularly effective acupuncture point for addressing digestive issues in children or young adults, as well as various respiratory problems, is located at the base of the left side of the thumbnail. This point can be treated quickly and effectively with a small prick of blood using acupuncture or a lancet pin.

we can see the same concept of radial nerve and lung meridian in eastern medicine

Western view the nerves in our body form different groups called trunks, and these trunks further split into divisions.

In the upper and middle trunks, the anterior divisions combine to create a bundle called the lateral cord.

The anterior division of the lower trunk forms another bundle known as the medial cord.

The posterior divisions from each of the three cords (lateral, medial, and posterior) join together to form the posterior cord.

These cords are named based on their position in relation to the axillary artery, which is a major blood vessel in the armpit region.

The radial nerve, like the axillary nerve, comes from the posterior cord, which is a group of nerves in our body.

It is often called the "Great Extensor Nerve" because it controls and provides movement to the extensor muscles of the elbow, wrist, and fingers. These muscles are responsible for extending or straightening these parts of the arm and hand.

In terms of sensation, the radial nerve also gives us the ability to feel things on the backside (dorsum) of our hand, specifically on the side of the hand that is closer to the thumb (radial side).

So, if you were to touch or feel something on that part of your hand, it would be due to the sensory signals transmitted by the radial nerve to the brain.

The median nerve arises from both the lateral and medial cords. It provides motor innervation to most of the flexor muscles in the forearm and the intrinsic muscles of the thumb (thenar muscles). Sensory innervation is received from the lateral (radial) 3 & 1/2 digits, which includes the thumb and the first 2 and 1/2 fingers.

From the eastern medicine view is the generally the same concept lung is yin meridian starting from brachial plexus to the thumb inside of the tumb nail meaning the yin meridian going up and large intestine meridian starting from index finger radial side down to the near the nose

This paring two meridian is the most important channel of breathing energy and covid and chronic disease more detail explain is coming

When we talk about "the first two and a half fingers on the same side of our hand," we are referring to the thumb, index finger, middle finger, and half of the ring finger on one side of our hand. These are the fingers that are connected to the median nerve. So, any sensation felt on these fingers, such as touch or temperature, is due to the signals transmitted by the median nerve.

Further more eastern medicine index finger is large intestine meridian middle finger is triple burner meridian and half of the ring finger on the side of our hand is heart the other small intestine meridian starting
Why so many symptom in covid in in pain of the hand and finger why the reason is the breathing line

Harold clinic

Why is the Lung Meridian First? The Lung Meridian is considered to be the first because between 1 am and 2 am, the heavenly energy opens, followed by the earthly energy at 2 am. The energy of the lungs begins to move at 3 am, starting with human breathing energy. At 5 am, the activity of the large intestine's energy takes place, allowing for the flow of qi or oxygen and the movement of blood.

What is Pain?

When it comes to pain, both Eastern and Western medicine have different perspectives. In Eastern medicine, it is believed that there is no need for painkillers. Instead, pain is seen as a natural response to certain disorders. By inserting acupuncture needles at the pain point, it helps to connect and balance the energy flow.

In Western medicine, pain is viewed as a phenomenon where individuals can feel physical sensations and pain in their own bodies. It is believed to originate from a top-down approach, focusing on the chemical composition of painkillers.

The concept of pain in Eastern medicine focuses on achieving wholeness rather than just eliminating the pain. It is seen as a sign that something inside the body is disconnected, and acupuncture works to connect the nerve pathways to restore balance.

By understanding the body's map of connections with qi and blood, Eastern medicine can determine the best diagnosis for pain relief based on which organ is affected. This holistic approach contrasts with the Western perspective that often relies on painkillers to address symptoms rather than treating the root cause of the pain.

Despite the origin in the brain, the passage states that the experience of unpleasantness and pain still persists. This suggests that individuals with mirror-touch experiences not only physically feel the sensations of others but also emotionally experience the pain associated with those sensations.

"Pain is the initial exclamation of 'OW!' followed by the instinctive urge to stop experiencing it. Pain feels genuine and evident, but it is actually an illusion that causes unfair suffering. The pain one feels in their index finger after a papercut is not truly located in the finger; it resides in the brain. Similar to other elements of the input-process-output model, the brain constructs a three-dimensional representation based on nerve signals from pain receptors in the finger.

These signals then initiate a series of subsequent signals..."

as the Japanese writer Haruki Murakami eloquently puts it: "pain is inevitable; suffering is optional." However, amidst life's trials, it can be easy to forget this wisdom.

These stories remind us that even in our ordinary lives, there is virtue in simply moving forward, one step at a time. It is a testament to the trying times we face that these stories seem to surround us today: from the struggles in Eastern Europe and the Middle East, to the unhoused individuals seeking shelter in tents and cars, and to the endurance of the sick in hospital emergency rooms, as well as the dedicated healthcare professionals who care for them.

"Pain" and "suffering" are deep and complex human experiences that can manifest physically, emotionally, mentally, and spiritually. Here's a brief overview of each term:

When pain signals are received by the body, they travel through the spinal cord and make their way to the brain, resulting in the perception of physical pain. Prior to the initial pain signal, cell damage caused by tissue injury triggers the release of cytokines and other neuropeptides, which are part of the inflammatory response, including the Substance P molecule. Once released, these molecules activate pain fibers responsible for transmitting the sensory experiences of physical pain from the body to the brain. These signals are then processed in the brain, providing information about the location of the injury, emotional significance, aversion, and motivation.

More scientific reason of pain by the book medical medium by Anthony William

A nerve is similar to a string of yarn with small root hairs hanging from it.

When the nerve is injured, the root hairs detach from the sides of the nerve sheath. Virus searches for these openings and attaches itself to them.

In simpler terms, the nerve sheath is like a protective layer around the nerve, while nerve myelination refers to the coating that helps nerve signals travel faster.

Virus make home in this nerve making it toxic feel pain

Harold clinic

Pain in western all related to brain but eastern medicine make it simple just the pain point(ashi point) that need treatment attention

So, pain is the basic treatment point directly. The healing journey of cancer pain is inevitable if you do not like chemotherapy, meaning pain is a natural healing response and signifies that your organ tissue is functioning correctly. In stage 3 or 4 cancer, pain may not be felt at all because all cells are completely toxic.

Genes and the environment

Genes and the environment both contribute to who we are and what we do. Are we destined to endure vulnerability to Covid due to our genes? The relationship between genes and viruses is complex.

Let's start with a simple question: Do you choose to wake up and go to Goodlife Fitness 4 Less or attend a yoga class with a mat? This decision can shed light on your genetic tendencies. Both genetic predisposition and defects in the immune system can influence the development of infections.

Considering that thousands of DNA variations are needed to explain height differences among individuals, finding a single gene that makes someone vulnerable to Covid seems unlikely. This highlights the complexity of genetic influences on physical traits.

In Eastern medicine, DNA variations are not well understood. It is believed that DNA is fixed at birth by our parents, while the environment plays a significant role in determining our health outcomes.

"Lonely Man of Faith" by Rabbi Joseph Soloveitchik, published in the 1960s. Soloveitchik observed that there are two accounts of creation in Genesis and argued that these represent the two opposing sides of our nature, referred to as Adam I and Adam II.

Adam I the external, résumé Adam.wants to build, create, produce, and discover things. He wants to have high status and win victories.
Adam Il is the internal Adam. Adam II wants to embody certain moral qualities.

Adam II wants to have a serene inner character, a quiet but solid sense of right and wrong not only to do good, but to be good. Adam II wants to love intimately, to sacrifice self in the service of others, to live in obedience to some transcendent truth, to have a cohesive inner soul that honors creation and one's own possibilities.

While Adam I wants to conquer the world, Adam II wants to obey a calling to serve the world. While Adam I is creative and savors his own accomplishments,
Adam II is humble and finds fulfillment in helping others.

Adam I seeks power and recognition, while Adam II seeks purpose and meaning in his actions. Despite their differences, both Adams face a constant inner struggle between their ambitions and values. Ultimately, Adam II's selfless nature sets him apart as a true leader,
while Adam I's selfish desires may lead to his own downfall.

Adam II sometimes renounces worldly success and status for the sake of some sacred purpose.
Adam II occasionally relinquishes material success and status in favor of a higher, more sacred calling.

Adam I asks how things work,
Adam II asks why things exist, and what the ultimate purpose of our existence is. While Adam I wants to explore and venture forth, Adam II prefers to return to his roots and appreciate the warmth of a family meal.
Adam I's motto is "Success," while Adam II views life as a moral drama and lives by the motto of "Charity, love, and redemption."

Soloveitchik argued that we are constantly torn between these two aspects of our selves. The outer, majestic Adam and the inner, humble Adam are never fully reconcilable, leading us to be stuck in a perpetual state of self-confrontation.

We are called to fulfill both personas and must master the art of living forever within the tension between these two natures.

The challenging part of this confrontation is that Adams I and II operate by different logics.

Adam I, the creating, building, and discovering Adam, lives by a straightforward utilitarian logic. It is the logic of economics - input leads to output, effort leads to reward, practice makes perfect, pursue self-interest, maximize your utility, and impress the world.

Adam II lives by an inverse logic. It's a moral logic, not an economic one. You have to give to receive. You have to surrender to something outside yourself to gain strength within yourself. You have to conquer your desire to get what you crave.

Success leads to the greatest failure, which is pride. Failure leads to the greatest success, which is humility and learning. In order to fulfill yourself, you have to forget yourself. In order to find yourself, you have to lose yourself.

"Adam II's moral core" involves recognizing and addressing our weaknesses, vulnerabilities, shortcomings, and areas for personal growth. Confronting these weaknesses, which are linked to the metal and water elements in Eastern philosophy, can make us more susceptible to viruses, stress, and infections.

Our society values the development of our external selves (Adam I) more than our inner selves (Adam II). The focus on building a successful career often neglects the importance of nurturing our inner lives.

The intense competition for success and admiration can consume us. Our consumer-driven culture encourages us to prioritize satisfying our desires, leading us to overlook the moral consequences of our daily decisions. Additionally, the constant bombardment of fast-paced and superficial communication can drown out the quieter inner voices.

Harold clinic of gene and environment

In a case study, a tall, healthy young man visited with shoulder pain. Despite being a 3rd-year student at Dalhousie University and regularly going to the gym for a six-pack like his friends, it was determined that heavy lifting could cause damage to his ligaments. Acupuncture was recommended for the broken tissue caused by heavy lifting, as it was not in line with his genetic makeup for muscle development.

What does that mean? I mean, when you do aerobic exercise, you need more oxygen than just for getting a six-pack, "Your genes are actually programmed for strong bones rather than a six-pack, You are already healthy and still growing, so don't follow trends. Normal gym workouts are enough to break a little sweat, but lifting too much weight can do more harm than good. If you go to the gym just for a six-pack, you will end up hurting yourself. Don't overdo it, listen to your gut - if it hurts, stop immediately. If you continue to exercise incorrectly, you can damage your connective tissue and have trouble with your shoulder and clavicle bones, which are connected to the lymphatic system for fighting off viruses. Pain in the muscles or away from the bone is not serious, but if it hurts near the bone, you need to take care of it. So, find your own workout plan - You can go hiking, play soccer, breathe in the forest air, or jump into the sea. That's what I recommend This book is for individuals like you, Adam 2, aimed at addressing your weaknesses and vulnerabilities to viruses. Confront your weaknesses, as being vulnerable to viruses, stress, and infections can increase the likelihood of experiencing more COVID symptoms and developing chronic diseases. On the other hand, Adam 2 can be free of viruses through detox and proper breathing, unlocking huge potential like most sports celebrities. Adam 2 is the type of person who loves movement, sports, and focus. What will you choose - losing your potential to a virus or achieving great success in what you love with the right information and direction?

Types of blood and viruses

Another method to investigate the relationship between blood types and viruses is through understanding the correlation between them. While some still believe in the 'blood-type personality theory,' there is a growing interest in the connection between blood type and diseases, rather than personality analysis. While blood type does not fully determine one's personality, it can give an indication of what diseases they may be predisposed to.

Professor Nakao Atsunori, from the Faculty of Medicine at Okayama University in Japan, stated in his book "A university professor explains the secrets of the human body like a lie," published last year, that individuals with blood type O are less likely to develop certain diseases compared to those with blood types A, B, and AB.

Professor Nakao referenced various international studies that suggest susceptibility to certain diseases based on blood type. A Swedish university study (2010) found that individuals with type A blood had a 1.2 times higher risk of developing stomach cancer compared to those with type O blood. Additionally, a paper from the U.S. National Cancer Institute in 2019 showed that individuals with type B blood had a 1.72 times higher risk of developing pancreatic cancer than those with type

O blood. Type B individuals also had a 1.21 times higher likelihood of developing type 2 diabetes.

Stroke, which has a high mortality rate as a single disease, is another condition that showed a correlation with blood type. Stroke is typically caused by sudden blockages or ruptures of blood vessels in the brain. Professor Nakao noted that individuals with blood type AB have the highest risk of developing stroke. According to a U.S. study published in 2014 on ABO blood type and stroke risk, individuals with type AB blood had a 1.83 times higher risk of stroke compared to those with type O blood. Another U.S. study also pointed towards this association.

In the same year, research also found that individuals with type AB blood are 1.82 times more likely to develop dementia than those with type O blood. One theory for why type O blood has the lowest risk of stroke is that it lacks antigens in the red blood cells, which may decrease the likelihood of blood clotting. Blood types are categorized based on these antigens, with type O blood being the only type without an antigen.

Individuals with type A, B, or AB blood have a higher risk of blood clot-related diseases due to poor blood clotting. Specifically, types A, B, and AB have a 1.25 times higher risk of heart attacks compared to type O. Additionally, these blood types have a 1.8 times higher risk of deep vein thrombosis, also known as economy class syndrome.

It is unclear why type O blood is associated with lower disease risk compared to other blood types, but it is important to note that individuals with type O blood have a higher mortality rate in cases of severe bleeding.

Harold Clinic

Through my many clinics, it has been discovered that individuals with type O blood have a higher heart rate and lower lung contraction rate, resulting in increased blood circulation (Adam 1). Conversely, individuals with type A, B, or AB blood have lower heart rates and higher lung contraction rates, which may lead to hypotension due to blood stagnation (Adam 2)

So, if you have blood type O, your body tends to be cool, whereas blood types A, B, and AB tend to make your body warmer. This is the opposite of the way daily life usually functions.

Further research discusses the 5-element 5-organ energy chart in Chapter 3, providing more detailed information on the relationship between each organ's energy levels.

Internal and external personalities and internal and external diseases are topics worth exploring. Often, a person's character differs inside and out, with these two aspects often appearing in contrast with each other. The concept of external and internal personalities remains relevant.

Some individuals may seem fragile externally, but in times of crisis, they exhibit unexpected inner strength. Conversely, others may project strength outwardly, but when faced with significant challenges, they may not demonstrate the same level of courage as their external persona suggests. It is true that we all have dual aspects to our character - external and internal, positive and negative - and they must be in balance.

This duality is also reflected in how diseases manifest within us. The healing process emphasizes addressing internal diseases rather than focusing solely on external symptoms. Finding the inner strength to fight the virus within is essential during the healing process, rather than being consumed by concerns over external scars or appearances.

Chronic Fatigue Syndrome

There are 5 types of fatigue of eastern medicine These types are combined and not separated by organ as in Western medicine. They are based on the Five Element Theory and are not familiar to the Western community. The first type is wood (liver)fatigue, which is related to an overwalk and can cause muscle pain, making it difficult to walk. If you have a wood constitution, you are likely to prefer using a car rather than walking. The second type of fatigue is stomach fatigue, which is linked to the spleen and can result from a sedentary lifestyle. It affects body fluids and can cause issues with blood circulation for those with an earth elemental constitution. Therefore, It is important to avoid being a couch potato and instead lead an active lifestyle.

The third type is water (kidney) fatigue, which occurs when one cannot stand for long periods of time and may result in collapsing to the ground.

The fourth fire (heart) affects the eye that is mostly abused, leading to blood itself issues. The fifth metal (lung) lowers oxygen levels, highlighting the importance of oxygen breathing exercises. This constitution lacks adequate oxygen, increasing the susceptibility to viral infections. My question is, which part of the information do you find beneficial based on your chronic fatigue? Remember, it is important not to be a couch potato in case of earth constitution; it can cause harm, so make sure to get up and go for a walk. However, my wife experiences muscle pain while walking, as she is more of a wood liver type. It's intriguing how some people are better suited for walking than others.

Similarly, there are individuals who tend to feel dizzy or fall down when standing up long time, known as the water kidney type. This is not a disease, but rather a genetic trait that needs to be managed to avoid accidents.

The last type of metal lung, which is dominant in certain individuals, requires more movement and exercise. Warming up through physical activity can facilitate detoxification through sweating, allowing for better oxygen intake. It's similar to how athletes optimize their performance by ensuring they breathe in the best quality oxygen.

In the case of this type of infection, it is not appropriate for Western medicine to confine patients with lung issues to a hospital bed. This is only a temporary solution. It is important to get outside and engage in exercise as soon as possible.

From the Western medicine perspective, chronic fatigue syndrome is viewed as a complex disorder.

Dr. Sarah Myhill explains her book "Chronic Fatigue Syndrome and Myalgic Encephalomyelitis " This condition is a complex and debilitating chronic illness characterized by extreme fatigue that does not improve with rest and can worsen with physical or mental activity. Individuals with ME/CFS often experience a variety of symptoms, such as post-exertional malaise, unrefreshing sleep, cognitive difficulties (commonly referred to as "brain fog"), muscle and joint pain, as well as other symptoms that can affect multiple body systems.

Case study

Mark is from Toronto and is in his 50s. He looks healthy on the outside and is a big guy. During his first meeting, he complained of neck pain.

However, during subsequent visits to the clinic, he also complained of chronic fatigue, anxiety, and sleep issues. One Saturday, he came in smelling of alcohol with a slightly red face.

> Me: Did you drink alcohol?
> Mark: Yes, I drink with my son every weekend.
> Me: How do you feel now?
> Mark: I feel all messed up, so I came to see you.

I was puzzled because Mark always appeared fine on the outside, yet there was no clear reason for his persistent tiredness. Further examination revealed that his breathing was inadequate, leading to inflammation building up inside I discovered gout in his big toes, which was describing his overall health.

Mark had previously tried acupuncture treatments, which had helped alleviate his pain and improve his body condition. However, i noticed that Mark's pulse was weak, and questioned why it did not meet expectations. Mark did not provide a clear answer.

Mark later explained that he had kidney issues, which caused his body fluids to deplete quickly. After receiving skull acupuncture treatment for clear the brain, his condition improved.

The diagnosis is the same, but the interesting thing is that he is big and physically healthy. As I insert the needle into Indang, also known as the third eye chakra located between the eyes, he tells me that he feels a strong vibe throughout his body when the needle is placed there. This demonstrates how breathing affects the pulse and the importance of acupuncture points in Indang, which represents the Lung function point and is the main route for breathing oxygen. The brain utilizes 40% of the oxygen, and the rest of the body also requires it for metabolism.

The Indang point acts as a port for delivering oxygen directly to the frontal lobe of the brain. Gout developing in the big toe is caused by acidic blood. According to meridian theory, the spleen meridian begins in the big toe and extends up to the chest through its yin channel. This represents the connection of yin energy from the earth in the big toes for blood circulation and the absorption of oxygen from cosmic sources through the fingers, particularly the thumb and first finger. This is a fundamental concept of meridian theory.. In Eastern medicine, one can assess the condition of their oxygen and blood by examining the thumb and big toe. Mark, who is experiencing pain in his big toe due to gout caused by uric acid, exhibits similar characteristics to kidney stones in the big toe, as both the kidney and spleen meridians pass through the big toe.. According to the book "Drop Acid" by David Perlmutter, MD, the levels of acid in the body can be influenced by problems like leaky gut inflammation or excessive alcohol consumption, resulting in the production of uric acid.

The beer belly is often the main culprit for health issues among many western men. It is crucial to understand how the body produces acidity, how it affects brain fog, and how it impacts the immune system. While wine and spirits may be different, this book suggests that beer is harmful for the gut. Why does beer matter so much? Because wheat is inherently cold in nature and contains toxic preservatives. Therefore, it is worse than you may realize due to its impact on gut health. The gut is the primary root cause of many health problems, including susceptibility to viruses.

The gut is connected to the lymphatic system and can damage your defense system by accumulating toxins in your blood.

It is important for Mark to generate heat to circulate or detox below the ATP level due to his genes and the natural aging process that leads to a slower metabolism and organ function. Drinking beer excessively can tire out the kidneys and harm the blood.

I have noticed many guys who replace regular meals with beer, which may provide temporary satisfaction but can be harmful in the long run. All of these issues stem from the gut, including diet and intestine health, as discussed in the upcoming chapters. Leaky gut, which damages the inner lining of the intestine, can lead to insulin resistance, inflammation, and other health issues.

A fat belly is a sign of an unhealthy body system, referred to as the lower Jao in the topic of functional medicine before. This includes the Kidney and two intestines that are affected by uric acid calcification. There are two meridians that run through the Kidney and Spleen in the big toes, providing scientific evidence that the left side of the big toe represents the kidney, while the right side represents the spleen.

Mark's case shows that energy levels are being depleted according to western medicine. When two-thirds of all energy produced are used for essential physiological processes, it highlights the crucial role of energy metabolism in sustaining life. Mark's case is an example of depleted energy production affecting basic bodily functions and causing chronic fatigue.

Moreover, a mitochondrial energy score of 0.6 or lower indicates compromised energy efficiency within mitochondria, which are responsible for energy production in cells. A score below 0.6 suggests that these cellular powerhouses are operating at less than 10% of their usual energy capacity. This can lead to anemia, reducing the blood's ability to carry oxygen, exacerbating fatigue, and causing the heart to work harder in chronic illnesses.

Available energy = Energy delivery - Energy expenditure

Lung and large intestine are paring organs

It is time for the paring of organ function

Lung and large intestine are paring organs and heart and small intestine are paring

Their relationship is very important.

It is vital to find out the root cause of COVID and chronic diseases using the paring concept

It is surprising to know the paring concept in 1930 in Western medicine, as the book "The Wisdom of the Body" by Dr. Walter Bradford Cannon Dr. Walter Bradford Cannon explores the organization of our bodies and addresses the fundamental question of whether our physiological systems are designed with a generous or narrowly limited structure. Dr. Cannon delves into the concept of the "margin of safety" in bodily structure and functions, highlighting the adaptive mechanisms and redundancies that allow our bodies to maintain stability and respond effectively to internal and external stressors. sheds light on the remarkable resilience and efficiency of the human body in safeguarding health and well-being.

Dr. Walter Bradford Cannon highlighted by drawing parallels between the design principles used in engineering and the adaptive mechanisms in the human body. He noted that, just as an engineer considers not only the expected weights and pressures that a structure must withstand when designing a bridge, the human body also incorporates a margin of safety beyond immediate demands.

This margin of safety allows for flexibility, resilience, and the capacity to respond to unexpected challenges or fluctuations without compromising overall stability. By paralleling engineering principles with the intricate design and function of the human body, Dr. Cannon underscores the remarkable efficiency and adaptability of our biological systems in maintaining homeostasis and ensuring optimal health.

In Eastern medicine, there is a more detailed pairing concept based on the law of motion that states energy is divided into 0, 2, 4, 8, 16, similar to a double division. The dynamic pairing of yin and yang means that lung yin brings down cosmic energy from the thumb, combining it with the large intestine yang energy for circulation of lung energy.

It is a law of nature. The first pairing is the Lung and large intestine, and the reason for this is that they correspond to the first natural energy cycle in a human body's function. Starting from the Lung during breathing time from 3 am to 5 am, and the large intestine during natural energy moving time from 5 am to 7 am. This is important because most covid and chronic diseases affect both organs, making them the root cause of all virus diseases. Recently, lung cancer and colon cancer have become the most incurable diseases nowadays. The reason they do not show real evidence is that most of the Western medical community does not consider this perspective. Therefore, I have tried to understand it from an Eastern medicine point of view combined with the lymphatic system in Western view. In Western medicine, the rate of colon cancer is dramatically increasing, becoming the second-highest cause of death after the pandemic. This was not the case before, as conditions such as Colorectal polyps, Crohn's disease, and Ulcerative colitis were more common. Some have found answers in certain genetic syndromes that increase the risk of developing colon cancer.

Another study suggests that diet may play a role in the risk of developing colon cancer, particularly high-fat, low-fiber diets and red meat consumption. Some research indicates that simply switching to a high-fiber diet may not decrease this risk, so the exact cause of the connection is still unclear. This information is gathered from various clinics and research studies.

Both the lung and the large intestine serve important functions in the body. It is of note that the large intestine is considered a primary cause of colon cancer. The large intestine is classified as a yang organ, meaning it is the first in line of action, and the lung is the second, which suggests that lung diseases may be a result of dysfunction in the large intestine. The harmonious paring function of the large intestine and the lung is crucial for the overall health by wisdom of the body that we are designed. The large intestine, as a yang organ, operates like a moving belt where all substances. Large intestine performs the important functions of absorbing nutrients and carrying out basic detoxification through its lymphatic system. Waste is constantly passing through the large intestine and being emptied from the body.

The lymphatic system illustrates how the colon is connected to other parts of the body. Lymphatic vessels from the anal canal travel alongside the middle rectal artery and drain into the internal iliac nodes near the internal iliac vessels. These nodes then connect to the common iliac nodes, which drain into the lateral aortic nodes. Additionally, lymphatic vessels from the rectum drain into pararectal nodes near the rectal muscles, then pass through the sigmoid mesocolon to reach the inferior mesenteric nodes, before continuing to the preaortic nodes. Lymphatics from the anus ultimately drain into the superficial perineum and scrotum, leading to the superficial inguinal nodes.

It is important to note that the anus and rectum are covered by lymphatic fluids, allowing lymph fluids to flow freely inside the large intestine. which help to naturally detoxify the body. When these areas fail to function properly, various symptoms such as constipation, diarrhea, and colon cancer can occur. The core issue is a compromised lymphatic system in the anus and rectum.

The lymphatic system plays a crucial role in picking up body waste by circulating through lymphatic vessels. I discovered that the small intestine produces the lymph fluids, and the large intestine circulates them, both being yang organs. The heart and lungs are yin organs that are more closely related to the blood, making it a bit more complicated. Proper functioning of the rectum in the large intestine is essential to support breathing, detoxification, and overall health.

General belief saying, nothing related to the small intestine and large intestine is connected to the lymphatic system. Follow your gut, as everything stems from the gut. I want to emphasize that the gut is the root cause, as it is where the lymphatic system is located. Without understanding this concept, we cannot effectively fight against the Covid virus. Nothing else can perform this function, which remains a mystery to Western medicine.

For instance, my father passed away at 87 in a peaceful manner. He appeared normal until a day before his passing when his breathing stopped and his anus muscles stop at the same time, leading to leaking poop in the bed calling it death. This highlights the importance of maintaining a healthy lymphatic system in the anus and rectum for optimal detoxification and overall health.

Breathing through the nose alone is not sufficient. The anus muscles must also work together to affect the overall function of detoxing the body. We consume a lot of food, whether it contains toxins or not, and the digestion process can produce toxins as well. If there is a strong flow of lymph fluids inside the body, it is okay. However, most people neglect the importance of this system.

My father reads many health books and practices himself daily forest breathing early in the morning, takes cold showers to care for his skin, avoids smoking and alcohol, and eats well. The best thing is to say goodbye peacefully without experiencing any pain.

Once again, nose breathing and anus muscle function must work together in harmony.

I can recall a situation from 30 years ago when my daughter had to visit a doctor multiple times for problems related to her large intestine, such as pain and digestion issues. She experienced frequent constipation and was prescribed medication to alleviate the symptoms. However, when she sought advice from a specialist, the root cause of the problem remained unidentified.

Meridian theory suggests that acupuncture can be effective for treating conditions related to the anus disease. Lung 6 is located on the inner side of the forearm, approximately halfway between the wrist crease and the elbow, but slightly closer to the elbow. For cough relief, the point known as Lieque (LU 7) is located on the radial side of the forearm, just above the styloid process of the radius, and 1.5 cun above the horizontal crease of the wrist, where moxibustion can also be applied. This indicates that the acupuncture points for addressing lung and large intestine issues are located in the arm, which is interconnected with the respiratory system through the fingers.

I once treated a patient who was dealing with urinary inconsistency, a common issue for women post-menopause. After examining her pulse and breathing, it was discovered that she had previously undergone a tonsillectomy and was lacking in energy. This weak breathing led to a weakening of the anus muscles.

For more in-depth information, please refer to Chapter 2 on treatment, which views the anus as a portal for heavenly energy that must be synchronized with breathing. This is in line with Western medicine practices like Kegel exercises.

The downward movement of your diaphragm puts pressure on your pelvic floor, which can make it challenging to do Kegel exercises while breathing, especially if your pelvic floor muscles are weak. To help with this, take a deep breath and relax your belly while exhaling any toxic air. Then, when you inhale, expand your belly and slowly and comfortably take in air. Focus on the sensation of air moving through your body and be mindful of how your breathing feels.

Anus breathing involves using the anal muscles to regulate the body, activating the lymphatic system and the essence of jing. Contracting and relaxing the anal muscles is key to accessing your inner strength and the invisible energy from the cosmos. While breathing, you can slightly close the anus muscle and hold your breath, counting from 1 to 10. The anus not only supports breathing but also enhances oxygen intake at a rate twice that of lung breathing, which is limited to the chest. Anus breathing aids in the invisible flow of inner lymph, working in conjunction with the lungs and large intestine to provide more energy for chronic fatigue patients and revitalize vital energy. Counting from 1 to 10, 1 to 50, and finally 1 to 100 can help clear out inner toxins that are released through exhalation and gas expelled through the throat.

Anal breathing is essential, so try to keep your anus slightly closed withholding your inhale breath as much as possible.

Harold Clinic

We place great emphasis on the importance of breathing through the nose. Inhaling through the nose and exhaling through either the mouth or nose is recommended, as nose breathing activates the parasympathetic nerve in the cervical spine, particularly between the fifth and seventh vertebrae. This is where the autonomic nerve of breathing and parasympathetic nerve pass through, making this location susceptible to viruses that cause tonsillitis.

It is called an autoimmune response that is designed to and must be cleaned and free from viruses.

Most breathing problems are inside the clavicle bone.

Now we are focusing more on oxygen breathing, including anus breathing and nose breathing together.

Simply breathe in, slightly close the anus, and hold the breath for as long as possible.

You can count from 1 to 10, 1 to 20, and more while slightly closing the anus, then release and contract rhythmically while counting.

This is the core treatment for all chronic diseases and oxygen breathing. More on this will be discussed in the next chapter on yoga oxygen breathing.

The human nose is lined with erectile tissue

We will discuss the nose, which is the first passage for breathing and any potential breathing issues. In Eastern medicine, the nose can be divided into four sections, extending from the eyebrows to the tip. The area between the eyebrows is associated with lung function, while the lower, concave portion of the nose corresponds to the heart. The middle section represents the spleen, and the area around the nostrils is linked to kidney function. This shows how each part of the nose is specifically connected to an organ. Meaning nose show your overall health condition the more shine the more oxygen in.

The lungs are said to reflect emotions and feelings of sadness, which are associated with the metal element. When a person slouches and fails to straighten their chest, it can indicate a negative mood. It is not just the nose and lungs involved in this, but also the immune system, skin, lymphatic system, tonsils, throat, and chest are all part of the broad concept of lung health in Eastern medicine. It is believed that all these systems are interconnected.

All of these mechanisms are expressed through your face. Have you ever wondered why the nose is in the center of the face? There is a reason for the facial design by a higher power, as it indicates the proper function of your inner organs being displayed on your face. The face is an expression of your inner energy.

Therefore, if someone has a shining nose, it means their breathing oxygen properly. However, if they have a runny nose or are stuck with a virus inside their nose, it indicates that something is wrong with their nose.

One interesting topic in western medicine that caught my attention is the connection between the nose and erectile tissue, as discussed in the book "Breath: The New Science of a Lost Art" by James Nestor. The interior of the nose is covered in erectile tissue, which is the same type of flesh that covers the penis, clitoris, and nipples. Noses can actually become erect as well. Within seconds, they can engorge with blood and become large and stiff. This happens because the nose is more closely connected to the genitals than any other organ; when one becomes aroused, the other responds. Some individuals may experience severe nasal erections simply from thinking about sex, resulting in difficulty breathing and uncontrollable sneezing, known as "honeymoon rhinitis."

As sexual stimulation decreases and the erectile tissue becomes flaccid, the nose will also become relaxed. Despite Kayser's discovery, many years passed before a good explanation was offered as to why the human nose is lined with erectile tissue or why the nostrils alternate in airflow. There were several theories proposed: some believed that this alternating airflow helped prevent bedsores by prompting the body to switch sides while sleeping. Others thought that cycling airflow protected the nose from respiratory infections and allergies, while some argued that it allowed for more efficient smelling of odors.

The right nostril acts as a gas pedal. When you primarily inhale through this channel, circulation speeds up, your body gets hotter, and.

When breathing through the right nostril, cortisol levels, blood pressure, and heart rate all increase. This is due to the activation of the sympathetic nervous system, also known as the "fight or flight" mechanism, which elevates the body's state of alertness and readiness.

Additionally, breathing through the right nostril sends more blood to the opposite hemisphere of the brain, specifically to the prefrontal cortex. This area of the brain is associated with logical decision-making, language, and computation. In contrast, inhaling through the left nostril acts as a brake system to the right nostril's accelerator.

Guiding this intricate respiratory process are the turbinates, six maze-like bones (three on each side) that begin at the opening of the nostrils and extend just below the eyes. The turbinate's, also known as nasal concha, resemble seashells and aid in filtering out impurities and preventing intruders.

The lower turbinates, located at the entrance of the nostrils, are covered in pulsing erectile tissue, which is then covered by a mucous membrane. This membrane filters out particles and pollutants and provides a moist and warm environment for breathing. The mucous membrane plays a vital role as the body's "first line of defense" against potential infections and irritations.

Constantly in motion, the mucus sweeps debris at a rate of approximately half an inch per minute or over 60 feet per day. Similar to a conveyor belt, it collects inhaled debris in the nose, transports the waste down the throat, and into the stomach. In the stomach, the waste is sterilized by stomach acid before being delivered to the intestines and eliminated from the body.

This conveyor belt does not run on its own. It is powered by millions of tiny structures called cilia, which look like hair. Similar to a field of wheat gently moving in the breeze, cilia move constantly with every breath, beating as many as 16 times per second.

The cilia near the nostrils move in a different pattern than those further inside, creating a coordinated wave that helps mucus flow deeper. These cilia have a strong grip that allows them to work against gravity. No matter the position of the head or nose, whether it is upside down or right-side up, the cilia keep pushing inwards and downwards.

One of the benefits of this process is that the sinuses produce a significant amount of nitric oxide, a molecule that is essential for improved blood circulation and oxygen delivery to cells. The quantity of nitric oxide in the body can greatly affect immune function, weight, circulation, mood, and sexual function. Drugs like sildenafil (better known as Viagra) work by releasing nitric oxide into the bloodstream, which helps open the capillaries in the genitals and other areas.

Harold Clinic

Eastern medicine refers to the ethereal incorporeal spirit that passes through the anus as the spirit is stimulated invisibly by oxygen breathing to the erectile tissue. As mentioned before, all are connected by design - nose function is not just for breathing but also brings cosmic energy to your inner body through the erectile tissue.

In terms of acupuncture, for most breathing issues, the needle is inserted in the concha, creating a more efficient flow of energy to the lungs. This book explains the science behind breathing very well.

Most deeper breathing issues occur in the concha, where viruses first affect the cilia, leading to mucus not flowing properly. Beets are a good food for increasing nitric oxide for better breathing.

By ensuring proper oxygen intake, ATP production in the blood can increase by 20 times. This is something I place a strong emphasis on.

Why is hair important? Because it is all connected to the lymphatic system. Hair functions by nourishing fluids in the body with body fluid. A more important thing is that it is a point of virus attack where they are able to settle. For example, in the eyelids, inside the nose, and small intestine cilia. In terms of nose hair, it is the trigger point of all breathing issues, meaning the first contact point of breathing, a unique formula of detox liquids and special tissue in it. This special tissue has many tiny blood vessels that are invisible, circulating every second, making it vulnerable to adapting to the outer air that we breathe. The tip of the nose needs special care. For example, for most breathing patients, inserting an acupuncture needle results in one drop of toxic blood coming out, and then they feel good and breathe fresh. Try it, but the tiny and complex blood vessels have a special job. When the needle is inserted, feeling a sharp pain is no problem, meaning the healing connection as a whole is working. Additionally, if you have an eye problem, try putting the needle in the eyelid hair. Eye problems are not just in the eye, but also a connecting point to the eye

Autoimmune disorders and Respiratory issues.

If you enjoy cycling or swimming in the pool, you may suddenly feel short of breath for just 5 seconds without breathing, causing panic. This is an example of an autoimmune issue that we have designed to not cause panic at all.

The reason for this issue is that the connection between nerves and blood is not working properly. There are many reasons for this, mainly caused by a virus, accident, or other factors that impact your immune function. This results in damage to the breathing nerve located in the back of the neck, connecting to the tonsils and ultimately to the brain's control of the autonomic nervous system.

When this circuit is not functioning properly, you may feel panic after just 3 seconds of not breathing, which is not normal.

When someone starts feeling short of breath and panics, the question that arises is whether the issue is related to an autoimmune disorder or simply a need to regulate breathing properly. The autoimmune response has the potential to disrupt communication within the brain, resulting in what is known as an autoimmune disorder.

Additionally, they had a runny nose which was very irritating. Unable to swallow due to excessive mucus, the runny nose persisted until medication was taken. The immune system's defense mechanisms seemed to be ineffective.

The study also looked at the connection between breathing and digestion. All bodily functions, including breathing, digestion, sweating, etc., are influenced by the immune system. This raises questions about why the immune system is unable to combat infections more effectively.

The accumulation of viruses over time suggests that the body is constantly fighting against infections since birth. However, some individuals respond quickly to these challenges while others take longer. This discrepancy raises the question of whether we are inadvertently acting against our own immune systems.

The negative energy you feel when someone cuts you off in traffic or wrongs you at work is the sympathetic system kicking in. In these situations, the body redirects blood flow from less vital organs, like the stomach and bladder, to the muscles and brain.

This causes the heart rate to increase, adrenaline to kick in, blood vessels to constrict, pupils to dilate, palms to sweat, and the mind to sharpen. Sympathetic states help reduce pain and prevent blood loss if we are injured. They make us more aggressive and alert, so we can react quickly in dangerous situations.

However, our bodies are designed to only remain in a heightened sympathetic state for short periods of time and only occasionally. While sympathetic stress can be activated quickly, it can take an hour or more to return to a state of relaxation and restoration. This is why food may be

After a stressful event, it can be difficult to digest why men may have difficulty with erections and women may struggle to reach orgasm when angry. For these reasons, it may seem strange and counterintuitive to voluntarily subject oneself to prolonged periods of extreme sympathetic stress on a daily basis. Why would one make oneself light-headed, anxious, and weak? Despite this, ancient cultures have developed and practiced breathing techniques for centuries that achieve just that., specifically focusing on the nerve auto immune system.

Eastern perspective on autoimmune dysfunction.

The spine, a long and flexible column of bones that protect the spinal cord, is divided into four sections: the cervical spine (neck), thoracic spine (upper and middle back), lumbar spine, and sacrum. Understanding autoimmune dysfunction is crucial, especially in the cervical spine where all functions related to the immune system, such as the parasympathetic nerve to the viscera, are concentrated. While this concept is not yet common in Western medicine, clinics and research have confirmed its validity and usefulness in treatment. Knowing which bone corresponds to specific functions, such as asthma, tonsils, and adenoids, provides valuable information for treatment. It is important to understand this detail for optimal health and well-being.

The cervical spine in the neck consists of 7 bones, with the upper 4 bones connecting to the liver, gallbladder, spleen, and stomach. The 4th bone is associated with the spleen and tonsils, while the lower 3 bones relate to the tonsils, adenoids, bronchial asthma, heart, lungs, thyroid, and mammary gland.

By using acupuncture to target specific points on these bones, it affects their function and can identify any underlying issues causing pain. The lower 3 bones of the cervical spine are crucial as they cover the autonomic nerve, which is essential in identifying early signs of autoimmune diseases.

It is important to check the connection between these 3 bones and the organs they interact with to address any potential issues. The remaining thoracic bones are associated with the sympathetic nerve and can be treated to alleviate upper and middle back discomfort.

Thoracic bones 1 and 2 are linked to heart and lung function, while bone 3 is related to external sensations and allergies. Bones 4, 5, and 6 impact lung health and breathing, with bone 3 influencing the upper limbs.

In the Peripheral Nervous System, nerves are categorized as either sensory (afferent) or motor (efferent). Sensory nerves carry information towards the CNS, while motor nerves transmit information away from the CNS. The PNS is further divided into two divisions: Somatic and Visceral.

The Somatic division relates to the muscles, skin, joints, and bones, primarily focusing on muscle function. The Visceral division is connected to internal organs and glands, such as the respiratory, digestive, urinary, circulatory, and reproductive systems, as well as certain sensory structures.

In simple terms, we are most concerned with the visceral division when it comes to breathing.

The Autonomic Nervous System (ANS), a part of the Peripheral Nervous System (PNS), acts as the "visceral efferent system" and consists of two subdivisions: sympathetic and parasympathetic.

The lymphatic vessels in the shoulder function similarly on both sides of the neck and clavicle, surrounding the shoulder and eventually leading to the brain. This is why the flow of lymph in the neck and shoulder is so important, as it can be a critical point for conditions like breast cancer or other severe tumors that invade the lymphatic system.

Western and eastern medicine may have slightly different perspectives, but the main concept is similar. Bringing them together offers more options for treatment, diagnosis, and healing. This concept is essential for advancing our understanding of the oxygen concept and uncovering the truth.

Harold Clinic

In regarding the nerve system Eastern Medicine offers more detailed explanations of specific points than Western Medicine when it comes to the autonomic nervous system. This information is valuable for treating breathing issues. For example, in the case of autoimmune diseases affecting breathing such as tonsillitis, focusing on the C4 and C5 points is crucial.

Before treating tonsillitis, I conduct an initial examination of the patient's neck muscles to locate any pain or abnormal thick tissue which may be affected by disease or viruses. In treating tonsillitis, I directly insert the needle below the jaw at the location of the tonsils, targeting the C4 and C5 points. This approach eliminates the need for surgery and focuses on the medulla oblongata at the base of the neck.

As noted by Bradford Cannon, excluding all sympathetic influences allows the vascular wall to modify the capacity of the vessels to hold body fluids, keeping them at a normal level to achieve balance.

Understanding terms such as mucus, serum, lymph

It is essential to have a clear understanding of viruses and the immune system in order to effectively treat both patients and yourself.

What is a cell membrane?

To clarify the importance of cell membranes, they are responsible for protecting cell integrity. Mucus also acts as a protective barrier on various body surfaces, especially the respiratory and digestive tracts.

I ask the chat box, "What is mucus and lymph?" The chatbot responds, "Mucus and lymph are both components of our body's defense mechanisms. Mucus acts as a physical barrier and helps trap pathogens and foreign substances, primarily in the respiratory and digestive tracts. On the other hand, lymph is a fluid that circulates throughout our lymphatic system, carrying immune cells and antibodies to fight infections and remove toxins from the body."

I inquire, "Is mucus and lymph coming from the small intestine?" The chatbot explains, "Mucus is primarily produced by specialized cells known as goblet cells. It is composed of water, mucus glycoproteins, antibodies, enzymes, and other substances that protect and lubricate the linings of the respiratory and digestive tracts."

Regarding lymph, the chatbot clarifies, "Lymph is a fluid derived from interstitial fluid. It contains white blood cells called lymphocytes, proteins, fats, and other molecules. Lymph is collected from tissues by lymphatic vessels and transported throughout the lymphatic system. It plays a vital role in immune defense, waste removal, and the transportation of important nutrients and hormones throughout the body."

I then ask, "Where are goblet cells located?" The chatbot explains, "Goblet cells are primarily found in the epithelial linings of various organs, particularly in the respiratory and digestive systems. They are abundant in the lining of the respiratory tract, including the nose, trachea (windpipe), and bronchi (airway tubes). Goblet cells help produce mucus that traps and removes dust, debris, and pathogens from the respiratory passages."

The digestive system includes goblet cells in the epithelial lining of the digestive tract, especially in the stomach, small intestine, and colon. This is important for digestion and breathing.

However, I am unclear about plasma, serum, and lymph fluids.

Plasma technology is based on the principle that matter changes state when energy is supplied to it. Solid becomes liquid, liquid becomes gas, and with more energy, gas becomes ionized and enters the plasma state, which is the fourth state of matter.

The term "serological" relates to the study of blood serum and its components, particularly in medical or scientific settings. Serology involves testing blood serum for markers like antibodies, antigens, and hormones to understand a person's health, immune response, and disease diagnosis.

Blood serum is the clear, yellowish fluid left after blood clots are removed. It contains proteins, electrolytes, hormones, antibodies, and other dissolved substances from blood plasma. Serum is a valuable specimen for diagnostic testing in medical labs because it reveals information about a person's health, immune response, and nutritional levels.

Serum is typically collected through blood centrifugation, where blood is spun at high speeds to separate its components.

Serum is the clearer, straw-colored liquid that rises to the top after centrifugation based on their densities.

Medical professionals utilize blood serum for a wide range of diagnostic tests, including measuring levels of glucose, cholesterol, liver enzymes, kidney function markers, electrolytes, and other substances that can provide insights into a person's health and assist in diagnosing certain medical conditions.

Serum and lymph fluids are both crucial components of the body's circulatory and immune systems, but they possess distinct characteristics and functions. Here are the key differences between serum and lymph fluids:

Serum:

- Serum is the clear, yellowish fluid that remains after blood has clotted and the clot has been removed.
- It is the liquid component of blood that does not contain blood cells or clotting factors.
- Serum contains various proteins, electrolytes, hormones, antibodies, and other substances dissolved in the blood plasma.
- Serum is collected through blood centrifugation and is used for diagnostic testing in medical laboratories to measure various substances and markers related to an individual's health status.

Lymph Fluids:

- Lymph fluid is a clear, colorless fluid that is derived from the interstitial fluid surrounding tissues.
- Lymph fluid is collected by lymphatic vessels and transported through the lymphatic system.
- Lymph fluid plays a crucial role in immune function, as it carries.

White blood cells, such as lymphocytes, and other immune cells throughout the body help to defend against infections. Lymph nodes, which are small structures located along the lymphatic vessels, filter and monitor the lymph fluid for pathogens and foreign particles.

In summary, serum is a component of blood that remains after clotting and contains various substances dissolved in blood plasma. Lymph fluid is a clear fluid derived from interstitial fluid that plays a key role in immune function and is transported through the lymphatic system. Serum is primarily used for diagnostic testing in medical laboratories, while lymph fluid is involved in the immune response and lymphatic circulation throughout the body.

Blood serum is an essential component in medical diagnostics and research, providing valuable information about a person's overall health and the functioning of various bodily systems. Another interesting aspect of research is on mucus from a western chemistry perspective.

One common chemical agent that helps prevent infection is mucus, also known as snot. It is produced not only in our noses but also lines our lungs, digestive system, and reproductive tracts. Mucus is a complex mixture of sugars, proteins, and DNA, with sticky proteins called mucins. The types of mucus produced vary depending on the location in our body. For example, airway mucus needs to be thinner and more easily penetrated compared to gut mucus due to the differing functions of the lungs and digestive system.

To create mucus at home, you will need 5 grams of pig mucin, 4 grams of salmon sperm DNA, 5 grams of salt, and some egg yolk.

Salmon sperm DNA and pig mucin may seem like unusual ingredients for many, especially if you are not involved in handling fish or swine. This is why it is important to consume fish for brain health and mucus production.

Mucus is just one of the powerful antimicrobial substances our body uses to fight off infections. In addition to mucus, enzymes play a key role in eliminating pathogens. These enzymes, which are proteins that speed up chemical reactions in the body, were named by German physiologist Wilhelm Kühne after the Greek word for yeast, as yeast aids in the fermentation of fruit into alcohol.

Most of the infection-fighting enzymes in our bodies are proteolytic, which means they break down other proteins. Interestingly, the same enzymes that help us digest food are also effective at breaking down bacterial components in the stomach.

In addition to these versatile digestive enzymes, our bodies produce enzymes that target bacterial biochemicals specifically. One example is lysozyme, which breaks down bacterial walls by targeting a chemical called peptidoglycan that holds bacteria together. Lysozyme is found in human breast milk, reducing the risk of diarrhea in infants, as well as in tears to prevent conjunctivitis. It is also abundant in the egg whites of chickens.

Aside from milk, hen eggs also contain lysozyme, which helps prevent bacterial infections. Eggs provide essential nutrition for the developing chick, making them susceptible to bacterial growth. If eggs are not refrigerated, lysozyme breaks down, leaving the egg vulnerable to infection.

Due to its easy accessibility, lysozyme was one of the first proteins to be extensively studied.

In addition to active processes that target and kill bacteria, we also use passive processes to deprive bacteria of nutrients. Pathogens need essential elements like carbon, hydrogen, oxygen, nitrogen, sulfur, phosphorus, potassium, sodium, magnesium, iron, calcium, manganese, zinc, cobalt, copper, and molybdenum to grow and survive, most of which are found in the human body.

However, the abundance of these nutrients increases our vulnerability to bacterial infections. Therefore, we have evolved to limit bacteria's access to these nutrients. In 1975, Eugene Weinberg introduced the term 'nutritional immunity' to describe how our cells prevent bacteria from obtaining our nutrients.

Iron is crucial for various biological processes. Humans mainly use iron in red blood cells to transport oxygen in the body. A lack of iron in one's diet can lead to fatigue and anemia. Similarly, bacteria require iron to metabolize sugars using oxygen. The level of free iron in the blood is closely regulated to prevent infections.

"Snot" refers to the mucus produced by the nose and sinuses. It plays a vital role in the respiratory system by trapping dust, bacteria, and other particles, humidifying the air we breathe, and protecting the delicate nasal tissues.

The color, consistency, and quantity of snot can vary based on factors such as hydration levels, allergies, infections, or irritants in the environment. While dealing with snot may not always be pleasant, its presence is a normal and essential part of the body's defense mechanisms.

In eastern medicine of body fluids

Body fluids are associated with specific organs combined not just one organ . Sweat originates from a combination of the heart and lungs, tears from the liver and kidneys, lung intestinal fluids from the spleen and large intestine, mouth fluids from the kidneys and spleen, stomach fluids from the liver and spleen, urine from the kidneys and bladder, and sperm from the kidneys and liver.

It is still unclear in clinical practice the distinctions between these body fluids. It is recommended to consume plenty of natural fruits to support digestion and immune function. However, based on this information, the focus should be on lymph fluids, which help protect against viruses. This book addresses the oxygen and lymphatic system, both of which are invisible and challenging to assess through lab tests

Virus

The master stated that in Eastern medicine, there is no clear concept of viruses.

We are not aware of the virus.

It makes no sense whatsoever.

Western medicine is widely regarded as the main approach for combating many viruses., which is why Eastern medicine is often perceived to be lagging. The Master explained that this is due to the lack of micro machines to observe viruses and the limited history of virus analysis. Eastern medicine takes a unique approach by focusing on the five basic organs. When a virus enters the body, symptoms are examined to identify which organ is affected and how it responds. For instance, in cases of food poisoning, the susceptibility to the virus varies among individuals based on the efficiency of their detox functions, such as the liver, stomach, small intestine, and large intestine.

Ten years ago, there were not many books available on viruses. However, now there are resources such as "Medical Medium" by Anthony William and Dr. Sarah Myhill's book "CFS AND MYALGIC ENCEPHALITIS" that focus on virus-related topics. Medical Medium Anthony William actively participates in podcasts, and his website contains a wealth of information. He has also published other books that include practical cases of viruses. One interesting point Anthony makes is that he believes autoimmune diseases are actually caused by viruses, rather than being separate conditions. This perspective may be worth considering.

Dr. Sarah's specific approach to understanding the virus, along with her new theory on graphing how it spreads, is extremely impressive.

In cases of molecular mimicry, when the immune system mounts a response against a foreign invader, antibodies or immune cells may also mistakenly target similar molecules present in the body's own cells or tissues. This can trigger an autoimmune response, where the immune system attacks healthy cells and tissues, leading to inflammation and damage. The connection between molecular mimicry and autoimmunity suggests that exposure to certain pathogens or environmental triggers with molecular similarities to self-antigens may contribute to the development of autoimmune diseases. Understanding these mechanisms can help researchers and healthcare professionals better comprehend the causes and triggers of autoimmune conditions and develop targeted treatments.

In cases of chronic infection, microbes create protective wrappings known as biofilms, which shield them from attacks. Researcher MacDonald has revealed that amyloid, a substance associated with many chronic diseases for years, may serve as a shield for microbes. This discovery could open up new treatment options for diseases linked to amyloid, suggesting it may be a marker for chronic inflammation caused by infection. Examples of biofilms include dental plaque, coated tongue, gut mucopolysaccharide, fibrin clots, and amyloid plaques found in the brain related to diseases like Alzheimer's. The term "shield for microbes" refers to a protective barrier or defense mechanism that prevents the entry or spread of microbes, such as bacteria, viruses, fungi, and parasites, which can cause infections or diseases.

Biofilms are communities of microorganisms that adhere to surfaces and produce a slimy, protective layer that helps them stick together and to surfaces. Examples of biofilms include dental plaque, which forms on teeth and can cause dental issues like cavities and gum disease. Another example is a coated tongue, where microorganisms form a layer on the surface of the tongue.

In the case of a beer belly, biofilms can form on mucopolysaccharides in the gut, which make up the mucus lining of the gastrointestinal tract. Biofilms can also form on fibrin clots, blood clots containing fibrin and platelets, and on amyloid plaques found in the brain, which are linked to diseases like Alzheimer's.

Microbes may switch between different forms to avoid the immune system's defenses. For instance, Borrelia, the infectious organism causing Lyme disease, alternates between the cell-wall-deficient 'L-form' and the dormant 'latent cyst' form. By encapsulating itself in the inactive cyst form, the spirochete can remain hidden in the host for long periods until some form of immune suppression triggers the cysts to open and the spirochetes to multiply.

The 'L-form' refers to a state where the microorganism lacks a cell wall, which is a protective outer layer found in many microorganisms. This absence of a cell wall can make the microorganism more resistant to certain antibiotics and can change its behavior and characteristics.

When a microorganism is described as "more resistant to certain antibiotics," it means that the microorganism has the ability to withstand the effects of specific antibiotics that are typically used to kill or inhibit its growth.

COVID-19 virus through the ACE2

Viruses can be categorized based on various characteristics or the similarity of their genes. However, it is difficult to precisely classify or name them due to their constant mutation. The mechanism of lung infection by the COVID-19 virus through the ACE2 receptor is first seen in Western medicine.

In Eastern medicine, Viruses can be differentiated by their symptoms and patterns of turbid dampness. Coating and mucus play a crucial role in the behavior of viruses. The viral genetic material is delicate and needs protection from being destroyed by other organisms seeking to defend themselves from infection. To safeguard their genes, viruses encase them in a protein coat. This coat protein influences viral transmission, including the ability of viruses to infect different cell types and their stability in the external environment. Enveloped viruses acquire an extra layer of protection from lipid coats obtained from the host cell's membrane during the exit process.

The presence of entry proteins allows close interaction between the virus and the cell, enabling the virus to inject its harmful materials. This process is akin to the velocity of a myelinated electrical energy pocket, with each virus functioning like a separate entity.

Substances known as entry proteins target molecules present on host cells. For example, SARS-CoV-2 targets the ACE2 receptor found on lung cells, influenza targets sialic acid, and RSV targets nucleolin. The specific location of these targeted molecules depends on the particular virus in question.

This targeting of cells within an organism is called tropism. RSV and influenza only target lung cells, leading to respiratory infections. However, ACE2 receptors are distributed throughout the body, potentially contributing to the severity of COVID-19. Once a virus enters the body, it can infect various types of cells.

SARS-CoV-2 has shown the ability to bind to ACE2 receptors in multiple species, including humans, rabbits, bats, and pangolins.

Influenza is another virus that can jump between species. Influenza binds to sialic acid in two different orientations, known as a2-3 and a2-6. Bird influenza viruses prefer the a2-3 orientation, while human influenza viruses target the a2-6 orientation.

A capsid is a structure utilized by viruses to hide from the host cells.

The immune system is adept at recognizing genetic material from organisms, acting as a danger signal that triggers a rapid response leading to the body's elimination of the infection. Since viruses aim to discreetly enter cells with their genetic material, they avoid activating the alarm system.

One way they evade the host's alarm system is by encasing their genetic material in a protein, effectively concealing it. Viruses utilize various levels of sophistication to achieve this, some simply wrapping it up like a cotton reel while others form structures composed of multiple repeats of the same protein, resembling a football.

The symptoms of viral diseases depend on the specific cells infected by the virus. If the virus replicates in the respiratory tract, symptoms like colds will result. If the virus replicates in the liver, it will cause hepatitis. Similarly, replicating in the gut leads to symptoms like diarrhea.

Viral diseases manifest in various ways, and some viruses, such as Ebola, cause disease by direct damage to cells. Viruses manipulate the life and death processes of infected cells to replicate and spread.

Normally, cells have a limited lifespan and undergo a controlled process of cell death known as apoptosis, involving the engulfing of the cell's contents. However, viruses need to spread beyond the infected cell. To achieve greater spread, some viruses induce a different type of cell death called necroptosis.

The contrast between the two types of cell death mirrors how viruses operate.

Stars die apoptosis is like a black hole - the cell collapses in on itself and nothing escapes, while necroptosis is like a supernova - the cell explodes, spreading its contents everywhere.

The Ebola virus causes supernova cell death by bursting the cells lining the blood vessels, leading to the characteristic hemorrhagic fever, with blood leaking from the body.

Cell damage caused by viruses can trigger an exaggerated immune response; the immune system, in trying to fight off the virus, can end up damaging surrounding cells.

Many of the symptoms we associate with an infection come from the immune system doing its job; for example, fever results from the body raising its temperature to kill off infections by cooking them.

However, if you are a virus looking to spread from an infected cell, this is not beneficial. To achieve a greater spread, some viruses induce a different type of cell death, known as necroptosis.

The difference between these two types of cell death can be compared to how stars die: apoptosis resembles a black hole, where the cell collapses inward and nothing can escape, while necroptosis is like a supernova, where the cell explodes, scattering its contents everywhere.

Harold Clinic

This is very informative information on virus development based on stages 1, 2, 3, and 4. Further details will be provided later.

It is evident that the two types of cell death that mirror how stars die are accepted by both Eastern and Western medicine.

Apoptosis is similar to a black hole - the cell implodes on itself and nothing can escape; while necroptosis is like a supernova - the cell bursts, spreading its contents everywhere. The speed of the spread depends on the oxygen levels, the movement of lymph fluids, and the body's ability to screen for any type of virus.

The most chronic cases often result from a lack of oxygen, leading to improper cell function in stage 3 which can ultimately progress uncontrollably to lymphoma, a very dangerous and incurable cancer. Eastern medicine offers a couple of treatment options, as discussed in chapter 2 on the Yamm treatment in clinical cases.

Acupuncture with moxa targets the core of the cancer, breaking it apart into small pieces that can be eliminated by the body, similar to a supernova. The development of cancer typically starts with small lumps that grow into tumors which then conglomerate into more toxic tumors by stage 4. This is a critical moment for cancer patients, often accompanied by severe pain.

The basic treatment for any virus involves the application of heat, as viruses typically seek out cooler locations to attach to receptors in the lungs. However, they do not thrive in hotter environments. Therefore, the primary treatment approach involves using moxa to apply heat directly to the affected area, as detailed in chapter 2. During the infection stage, The virus cells are quickly destroyed as the lymph fluids leak abundantly, regenerating the immune function to restart.

During the healing stage, the process involves destroying the core virus that coats many layers of cells inward, causing it to divide and explode outward into pieces for the virus survivor. Once again, the virus is sensitive to heat and detaches from the human bloodline, feeding on toxic blood. This creates a killing spree of colonized viruses, but it is a natural healing process in Eastern medicine.

This process involves breaking the coating of the virus cluster using moxa to regenerate the lymphatic system and restore normal lymph circulation, which is essential for natural healing. The lymphatic system plays a crucial role in fighting off viruses and antibiotics.

Virus and antibiotic

Antibiotic resistance occurs when bacteria or other microorganisms change in response to the use of antibiotics, making the drugs less effective or ineffective in treating infections caused by these resistant microorganisms. In the context of antibiotic resistance, the resistant microorganism may have genetic mutations or mechanisms that allow it to survive the presence of certain antibiotics. This can make it challenging to treat infections caused by resistant microorganisms as standard antibiotics may no longer be effective against them.

The development of antibiotic resistance is a significant concern in healthcare as it can lead to prolonged illnesses, increased healthcare costs, and in some cases, treatment failures. Addressing antibiotic resistance is crucial to ensuring effective treatment of infections and preventing the spread of resistant strains.

In order to combat resistance, it is crucial to use antibiotics carefully, implement infection prevention measures, and develop new strategies to fight against resistant microorganisms.

On the other hand, the "latent cyst" form is a dormant and inactive state that the microorganism can enter. In this state, the microorganism is not actively reproducing or causing symptoms, but it has the potential to reactivate and resume its normal activities when conditions become more favorable.

This description indicates that the microorganism has the ability to switch between these two distinct forms depending on its environment and internal conditions. Understanding these transitions is essential for studying the biology and behavior of the microorganism and may have implications for developing treatment strategies to target or control its different forms.

Allergic reactions and infectious reactions may be a result of the virus hiding in the immune system and brain, preventing it from appearing in the bloodstream, making it challenging to measure the total viral load. However, this is not significantly important for practical purposes. The only difference between allergy reactions and infectious reactions is the quantity of antigens (the number of microbes) and the immune system's response to them.

One can view this as a spectrum of activity, ranging from the normal person with appropriate immune reactions, followed by the slightly sensitive, mildly allergic person, and finally, the highly sensitive person.

Quorum Sensing

The next big thing is quorum sensing, which is crucial for understanding how viruses cause infections. Viruses communicate with each other in a much smarter way than we realize. It is essential to have a basic understanding of this communication in order to comprehend why vaccines may not always be effective. Viruses possess information about vaccines, allowing them to adapt and survive. Therefore, it is important to protect oneself from viruses by boosting the respiratory and digestive systems.

The next big thing is quorum sensing, which involves understanding how viruses communicate with each other in order to infect. Viruses are smarter than we think, and it is crucial to have basic knowledge of how they interact to understand why vaccines may not always work effectively. Viruses have the ability to adapt and survive, making it necessary to protect yourself by maintaining proper respiratory and digestive health.

Quorum sensing, known as "A Small World After All," is a concept encoded in the DNA of bacteria. When bacteria are allowed to multiply for one hundred generations, the encoded information remains intact without any mutations. This demonstrates how bacteria can act as information time capsules, preserving knowledge for future generations.

Bacteria in our bodies can choose to either remain solitary and vulnerable to attacks from the immune system and antibiotics, or to form biofilms and increase their chances of survival. Biofilms are complex structures made up of polysaccharides, recycled DNA, and materials from deceased bacteria. These biofilms provide a collective defense mechanism for bacterial cells, allowing them to thrive in challenging environments.

As time passes, bacterial cells within biofilms will begin to interact with each other in unique ways, further enhancing their ability to survive and thrive.

Bacteria communicate through a chemical process known as quorum sensing, by releasing molecules that act as messages detected by nearby bacteria via nanotubes. These nanotubes have been found to operate between B. subtilis, Staphylococcus aureus, and Escherichia coli across different species.

Quorum sensing can occur within a single bacterial species as well as between different species. Bacteria use quorum sensing to coordinate behaviors such as virulence, antibiotic resistance, and biofilm formation. Gürol M. Süel and his team at the University of California San Diego have extensively studied long-range communication in biofilms.

They have observed waves of charged ions traveling through the biofilm to coordinate bacterial metabolic activity in various regions. Süel explained, "Just like neurons in our brain, bacteria use ion channels to communicate through electrical signals."

Bacteria in biofilms play a role in many chronic diseases and are highly resistant to drugs. Scientists from MIT recently discovered two strains of bacteria, each resistant to a different antibiotic, protecting one another in an environment with both drugs. These findings enhance our understanding of mutualism, a phenomenon usually associated with larger animals, where different species collaborate.

Bacteria benefit from their interactions with each other, leading to cross-protection that helps them form drug-resistant communities. Since 1983, Roberto Kolter, a professor of microbiology and immunobiology at Harvard Medical School, has headed a laboratory that has been studying these phenomena. Kolter has noted that under the microscope, the remarkable collective intelligence of bacteria is revealed in a visually stunning way. The imagery from the lab, featured in the exhibition "World in a Drop" at the Harvard Museum of Natural History, showcases this beauty.

Based on these and other related studies, many prominent cognitive scientists have concluded that communities of bacteria within biofilms appear to function as a microbial brain. Quorum sensing in bacteria refers to a mechanism that enables bacterial cells to communicate with each other and coordinate their behaviors based on population density. This process involves the production and detection of signaling molecules, also known as autoinducers, which are released into the surrounding environment by bacteria.

Once the concentration of these signaling molecules reaches a certain threshold, it signals that the bacterial population has reached a critical mass. At this point, the bacteria can detect and respond to the presence of the signaling molecules, leading to specific gene expression and coordinated behaviors. Quorum sensing allows bacteria to synchronize their activities, such as forming biofilms, producing virulence factors, releasing enzymes, or coordinating collective behaviors.

Behaviors are often essential for bacterial survival, pathogenesis, and colonization of hosts. Chronic viral infections have taught me a great deal about the work of Dr. Martin Lerner. I believe it might be more of an allergic reaction to the virus rather than simply a matter of total viral load.

Low levels of antigens pose no threat to the body and typically result in no symptoms. Moderate levels of antigens and high levels of antigens, such as with pneumonia, can present a modest threat to the body. In these cases, the immune system is alerted and appropriately activated. Severe symptoms may occur with high levels of antigens, potentially becoming life-threatening.

The response of a slightly sensitive, mildly allergic person, which accounts for 38% of the population, is as follows: low levels of antigens do not pose a threat, while moderate and high levels of antigens, like pneumonia, may present a modest threat, with the immune system being appropriately activated. Symptoms of allergies, such as catarrh, cough, asthma, headache, Irritable Bowel Syndrome (IBS), and arthritis, may be experienced.

Catarrh, cough, and asthma are all respiratory conditions, but they present with different symptoms and have distinct characteristics:

Catarrh (Mucus Build-Up): Catarrh refers to an excess production or build-up of mucus in the respiratory tract, typically in the nose or throat. It is often associated with colds, allergies, or other respiratory infections. Symptoms of catarrh can include a runny or blocked nose, coughing, throat irritation, and post-nasal drip. Treatment for catarrh often focuses on addressing the underlying cause, such as treating the infection.

Infection or managing allergies may involve therapies to help reduce mucus production and alleviate symptoms. A cough is a reflex action that helps clear the airways of irritants, excess mucus, or foreign particles. Coughs can be acute (lasting for a few weeks) or chronic (lasting longer than eight weeks). Common causes of cough include respiratory infections, allergies, asthma, or irritants such as smoke or pollution. Treatment for a cough depends on the underlying cause and may include addressing any infection, managing allergies, or using cough suppressants or expectorants to alleviate symptoms.

Asthma is a chronic respiratory condition characterized by inflammation and narrowing of the airways, leading to symptoms such as wheezing, shortness of breath, chest tightness, and coughing. Asthma symptoms can range from mild to severe and can be triggered by various factors, including allergens, respiratory infections, exercise, or exposure to irritants. Treatment for asthma typically involves using medications to manage inflammation and bronchoconstriction, as well as identifying and avoiding triggers to prevent asthma attacks.

Bronchoconstriction is a term used to describe the narrowing of the airway passages in the lungs, specifically the bronchi and bronchioles. This narrowing is typically caused by the tightening of the smooth muscle surrounding the airways, leading to restricted airflow and making breathing more difficult. Bronchoconstriction is a common feature of conditions such as asthma, where triggers such as allergens, irritants, cold air, or exercise can lead to inflammation and the tightening of the muscles around.

The airways can become constricted, leading to symptoms such as wheezing, coughing, shortness of breath, and chest tightness.

Treatment for bronchoconstriction often involves bronchodilator medications, which help relax the muscles around the airways, allowing for improved airflow. These medications can be administered through inhalers or nebulizers and are used to provide quick relief during asthma attacks or to manage symptoms of conditions characterized by bronchoconstriction.

Food antigens can be transferred into breast milk, and the baby's immune system may accept them as normal. Similarly, gut microbes can begin to be inoculated even before birth, possibly transferring across the placenta while the baby is in the womb and then undergoing further colonization during birth. The first 24 hours after birth are critical for this immune education to occur. These microbes are then nourished by friendly bacteria found in human breast milk, eventually colonizing the gut with the mother's bacteria. In its flexible learning state, the baby's immune system considers this normal.

The idea that "the flora begins to be inoculated even across the placenta while in utero" implies that the establishment of the body's microbial communities may start before birth, with microbes possibly being transferred from the mother to the developing fetus through the placental barrier during pregnancy.

The placenta, an organ that forms during pregnancy, facilitates the exchange of nutrients, waste, and gases between the mother and the developing fetus. While traditionally considered a sterile environment, current research suggests otherwise.

The placenta may not be entirely free of microbes, and a transfer of microorganisms from the mother to the fetus could potentially take place. This process, known as vertical transmission, may introduce beneficial microbes from the mother to the developing fetus. It could potentially help in priming the infant's immune system and shaping their early microbial colonization. The transmission of maternal microbes across the placenta is an active area of research that could have implications for understanding the development of the infant microbiome and its effects on health and immunity.

The term "inoculate" refers to introducing a microorganism (like a bacterium, virus, or other pathogen) into a host to stimulate the immune system and provide protection against future infections. Inoculation can also refer to introducing a substance, such as a vaccine, to generate immunity against specific diseases.

In the field of microbiology and immunology, inoculation is commonly used to establish microbial cultures in laboratory settings for research, diagnostics, or vaccine production. By inoculating a culture medium with a particular microorganism, researchers can study its growth, characteristics, and interactions in a controlled environment.

Regarding vaccination, inoculation involves administering a vaccine containing weakened or killed pathogens or their components to stimulate the body's immune response. This exposure allows the immune system to recognize and remember the pathogen, creating a "memory" that helps the body mount a rapid and effective immune response upon subsequent encounters with the same pathogen.

In general, inoculation plays a critical role in science, medicine, and public health by providing protection against infectious diseases.

Advancing our understanding of microbial biology and immune responses, intentional introduction of microorganisms or vaccines contributes to boosting immunity and preventing diseases in laboratory and clinical settings.

It is widely known that 90 percent of the immune system is linked to the gut. The mature cells at the frontline have the ability to distinguish between what they should and should not react to. Immature immune cells are released daily from the bone marrow into the bloodstream, where they learn from the mature cells at the frontline, primarily located in the gut. These immature cells learn to adapt to the current situation and as they mature, they also acquire immune memory which is passed down through generations, maintaining ongoing immune tolerance to gut microbes and food. This explains why the immune system can usually ignore these antigens and not react to them as if they were viruses. From infancy to adulthood, individuals have learned to do so.

The immune system's ability to regulate and maintain tolerance to gut microbes and food antigens is vital for overall health and immune function. By developing and upholding immune tolerance to these usually harmless elements, the immune system can concentrate its resources on combating true threats, such as pathogens, without triggering unnecessary immune responses to beneficial microbes or dietary components.

In the context of antibiotics, a high dose of these medications can have an impact on the immune system. Antibiotics are substances used to eliminate or restrain the growth of bacteria, which in certain instances, may also influence the body's immune response. High doses of antibiotics can alter the composition of the gut microbiota, which has a crucial function in regulating immune function and maintaining immune tolerance.

Exposure to high doses of antibiotics can upset the balance of gut bacteria, which can affect the immune system. This imbalance may make it difficult for the immune system to differentiate between harmful and harmless substances, potentially leading to immune system problems and increased risk of infections or inflammation.

Our immune system is designed to recognize and spare our own cells, just like other biological systems do. It needs signals to determine what is safe to interact with.

Too much inflammation from fighting infections can also be harmful. The immune system needs the right amount of inflammation for optimal health, rather than being in a constant state of battle.

Fat and certain tissues are crucial for the immune system to function properly. Fat is important for supporting immune cells, while bone marrow is essential for producing new immune cells.

Harold Clinic

viruses are much more complex than we previously thought, as they have the ability to communicate with each other in three-dimensional ways.

They survive by finding food within your body and locating the optimal location to thrive on fat, meaning viruses rob your nutrition by tapping into the pure blood vessels and using your oxygen to multiply for their survival. This causes toxicity to you, but for the viruses themselves, it is why they can be so damaging to your basic defense system.

We only rely on vaccines that the virus is already immune to, meaning they know how to adapt and depend on their own survival tactics. This is why COVID and chronic patients are growing dramatically in need of help.

Now, the responsibility is on your shoulders. Start with the basic principle of eating natural foods for your gut and focus on proper oxygen breathing.

But we only depend on the vaccine that virus already immune meaning they know how to move how to depend on their own

That is why covid and chronic patients growing dramatically to need help

Now all matter is on your shoulder starting basic principle eat natural food for your gut oxygen breathing second

3rd Brain: Skin

Skin is considered the third brain of the body. The Master explained that by regulating the body's temperature, most diseases can be cured. I don't fully understand what this means. It's actually quite simple: if your genes make you a "hot" type of person, then you should seek cold treatments. On the other hand, if your genes make you a "cold" type of person, you should seek hot therapy.

Our bodies operate at their best when there is a balance of hot and cold, all working together with the five organs. In simple terms, the heart and liver represent heat and warmth, while the lungs and kidneys function in opposition. The balance between these two opposing forces creates basic body energy. How well the body can harmonize and balance these forces determines whether a person is healthy or sick.

In Eastern medicine, cold and cool are considered medically distinct. Clear cold is similar to cold weather, while cool is the body's internal response to cold, indicating an internal condition. Cold refers to the external temperature of the atmosphere, whereas cool pertains to the internal temperature of the body responding to the atmosphere. Each person responds differently based on their body condition, meaning some may embrace the cold weather while others may catch a cold.

The topic of skin is viewed as more than just an external issue; it is now considered as an organ that communicates with the brain. Recently, the skin has been referred to as the 'third brain,' with the gut forming the 'second brain' through the gut-brain axis and gut bacteria. With a surface area of 2m square and weighing 5kg, the skin is the largest organ in our body. Therefore, proper skin care is essential for a longer and healthier lifespan, leading to a more youthful appearance.

As we age, the battle against dryness becomes more significant. Human life began in water, and we evolved from the sea. Our reliance on moisture is evident from the moment sperm and egg meet through swimming, to the growth of the fetus in amniotic fluid. To maintain a youthful appearance and sharp mind as we age, it is crucial to diligently apply sunscreen and moisturizer. Protecting the skin is essential for brain health.

Medicine has advanced through groundbreaking research, such as the discovery of induced pluripotent stem cells. Professor Shinya Yamanaka from Kyoto University in Japan successfully reverted fully grown adult skin cells back to the embryonic stage by injecting specific genes. This discovery challenged the common belief that aged cells could never regain their youth. Currently, induced pluripotent stem cells are used in therapies where new cells created from a patient are injected into damaged tissues and cells.

A study published in a U.S. psychiatry journal in the 2000s revealed that the condition of the skin can impact cognitive brain function. The study compared 80 patients with chronic skin conditions like eczema and atopic dermatitis to a control group of 80 healthy individuals. It was found that patients with skin conditions had lower scores in language memory and attention. This study suggested for the first time that the condition of the skin can affect cognitive function.

Not only do external factors influence brain function, but they also impact cognitive functioning. Consequently, there has been a growing awareness that improving cognitive function should be considered in the treatment of chronic skin conditions. Studies on the relationship between the skin and the brain have revealed important connections, such as "the more severe the dermatitis, the greater the risk of sleep disorders leading to cognitive impairment," "chronic dermatitis increases the likelihood of depression," and "acne impairs learning ability."

A recent European dermatology journal has published intriguing research. In this study, 200 elderly individuals over the age of 65 were divided into two groups. One group applied moisturizing lotion twice a day to keep their skin moist for six months, while the other group did not. Three years later, when their cognitive function was assessed, it was discovered that the group using moisturizer had lower skin moisture loss and better cognitive function. The research suggests that diligently applying moisturizing cream can delay cognitive decline in the elderly. Studies have shown that properly moisturizing the skin reduces inflammation markers associated with aging, while skin dryness and poor condition elevate serum inflammatory cytokines, supporting the cognitive benefits of moisturizers.

Understanding the basic skin infection process is crucial. The formation of plaques happens when immune cells enter the skin from the bloodstream and send incorrect signals to the skin cells. These chemical signals, such as the molecule TNF, cause skin cells to divide too quickly and promote the growth of blood vessels towards the skin's surface. These findings highlight the impact of moisturizers on cognitive function and the importance of skin health in overall well-being.

Division in the skin can also lead to an increase in the number of blood vessels that extend and branch towards the edges of the skin. The skin is one of the most efficient ways for the body to eliminate toxins, primarily detoxifying without causing scarring. However, situations like a chickenpox infection can result in scratching that leads to the formation of scars and discoloration in the areas where blisters appear.

The skin is composed of two layers: the epidermis (the upper layer exposed to the air) and the dermis (the lower layer containing blood vessels). In the case of a psoriasis plaque, the top layer of the skin becomes thicker due to faster cell multiplication compared to healthy skin, with an accumulation of dead skin leading to flaking off. The increased number of blood vessels running through the skin causes it to appear red, making it prone to bleeding if the flakes are scratched away.

If the skin can absorb medications more effectively than swallowing, what happens when lotions or cosmetics filled with toxic chemicals are applied? Or when hair dye, gasoline, or toxic cleaning products are used without protective gloves?

Eastern medicine for the skin

In Eastern medicine, the meridian systems are divided into three levels: superficial, mid-level, and deep, which correspond to exterior, half-exterior, and interior level.

Superficial levels consist of 12 cutaneous regions, including the skin and muscles, as well as superficial luo-connecting vessels and 12 sinew channels

Mid-levels include 1/16 luo-connecting vessels), external pathways of the 12 primary channels, external pathways of the 12 divergent channels, and eight extraordinary vessels.

Deep levels encompass the internal pathways of the 12 primary channels (related to zangfu-Organs) and the internal pathways of the 12 divergent channels.

Each primary channel, along with its corresponding secondary channels, forms a complex and multi-layered organizational unit known as a "system." These systems establish various relationships and connections with each other and with the eight extraordinary vessels, supporting harmonious regulation within the body.

Wei qi flows circulate outside the mai (the channels and vessels) and also along the channel pathways, particularly in the space between the skin and muscles known as the cou li.

The cou li, often mistakenly translated as "pores," are actually the striae or compartments between the skin and muscles. They act as gateways for the entry and exit of Qi and fluids and provide protection against the invasion of Exterior pathogenic factors.

Harold Clinic

I enjoy emphasizing the importance of skin breathing and skin treatment. Many traditional practices, like those of the people of Finland and others, include saunas and ice baths. Athletes often use ice baths to alleviate pain.

Inflammation and recovery times can be improved through ice baths. However, staying in an ice bath for too long can lead to hypothermia and death. When done at the right temperature for the appropriate duration, ice baths offer numerous health benefits. These benefits include elevating endorphins, strengthening the immune system, reducing inflammation, boosting metabolism, facilitating weight loss, improving circulation, and stimulating the vagus nerve, which triggers the body's deep relaxation response.

Ice baths also increase focus, mental clarity, and the production of dopamine, the pleasure neurotransmitter. Activating the "brown fat" located between the shoulder blades generates heat and energy. For example, during a month-long stay in a winter cabin, starting each day with an invigorating ice-cold shower, completely replacing the need for a cup of coffee.

Scientific evidence supports cold therapy methods such as cold-water swimming, cold showers, cold plunges, and cryotherapy, which are available at various centers across the country.

Healthier skin requires increased oxygen intake. Oxygen is transported through the bloodstream via Qi (life force) to provide an effective cure. Just breathing in regular air without oxygen is not effective and cannot provide a cure. Oxygen works in conjunction with the autonomic nervous system and the parasympathetic nervous system, but accidents, stress, and other factors can interfere with this process.

Breathing in oxygen not only prevents viruses from spreading or disappearing but also activates lymph and blood circulation, allowing hemoglobin to carry optimal amounts of oxygen to the glands for their proper functioning. Optimal functioning of mucus and the white blood cells in the lymphatic system are interconnected. Without a healthy lymphatic system, viruses can easily infiltrate the body. The concept of wind can be explained as the fluctuation in air flavor sensed by the left arm and the complex emotions experienced by the right side.

Case study

Joint tuberculosis, a disease that was previously thought to be incurable like a beehive, was cured with a hot-cold method. Professor Goto Yukimashi from Japan, who had fallen into despair as his bones, flesh, and skin were pierced with holes like a beehive from malignant joint tuberculosis, healed completely with a treatment involving hot towels and ice packs alternately on the affected area.

He would repeatedly wrap the affected area with a hot towel until it became hot, then cool it with ice cubes (cold) to cure the disease. While it may not be a quick fix after just one or two tries, he was able to cure what had not improved in 3-4 years at the hospital in just two and a half months, making one wonder how such a simple method, almost as foolish as it may seem, could actually be the best treatment for humanity.

Using heat properly can cure all illnesses. Professor Goto is pleased to have become a natural therapist after this experience as an engineering doctor.

The skin also provides vitality, so when doing saunas, alternately applying cold and hot water from the thumb, where the lung meridians flow, to the shoulder, and from the pinky finger, where the cardiac nerves flow, to the shoulder, can be very helpful. Just like watering leaves of a tree every day to keep plants alive, supplying oxygen through fingertip massages and the nerves passing through the fingertips to the shoulder with cold water can be a good respiratory therapy.

"If you keep your head cool and your feet warm, you can laugh at all ailments." This quote comes from the renowned 18th-century Dutch philosopher and physician, Boerhaave. According to his teachings, simply rubbing your hands together and elevating your feet can help cure any illness.

Each cancer stage

The connection between gut health and breast cancer in women is significant. It is essential for women to regularly perform self-examinations for lumps before the cancer reaches an advanced stage and to consult a doctor promptly if any are detected. Women are particularly susceptible to blood-related issues, so even a minor infection can become a serious concern. Therefore, consistently monitoring for lumps is vital. In this context, I will present the stages of both this type of cancer and lung cancer, drawing from my own research.

The immune system is our standing army - keep it standing and not fighting!

The immune system has a difficult job to do. It has to recognize those things which are good for us (such as food) from things that are bad for us (such a unfriendly microbes).

Sometimes it has to swing into action to fight infection this involves inflammation (pain, heat, swelling, redness and loss of function, Although short-term inflammation is vital to prevent death from infection, it is a dangerous tool - there is great potential for damage to self through

Breast and peritoneal cancer are serious medical conditions that require prompt and thorough treatment.

The stages of breast cancer are as follows:

- Stage 0 is preinvasive (DCIS).
- Stage 1 refers to a tumor that is less than 2 centimeters and contained within the breast.
- Stage 2 describes a larger tumor that is confined to the breast or involves some axillary lymph nodes.
- Stage 3 is a locally advanced tumor that has spread to the breast skin or chest muscle, or involves several lymph nodes in the armpit or above/below the collarbone.
- Stage 4 indicates that the cancer has spread to other areas of the body beyond the breast and lymph nodes. This stage is also known as metastatic breast cancer.

Approximately 90 percent of sporadic and hereditary epithelial cancers originate from the cells that cover the ovaries and line the fallopian tubes. Peritoneal cancer contains similar epithelial cells. Peritoneal cancer, also known as primary peritoneal cancer, is a type of cancer that originates in the peritoneum. The peritoneum is a thin, transparent sheet of tissue that lines the inner walls of the abdomen and covers the organs within it, such as the stomach, liver, and intestines.

Peritoneal cancer is similar to ovarian cancer in terms of its symptoms, diagnosis, and treatment because both types of cancer can develop from the same type of cells in the peritoneum. However, peritoneal cancer specifically refers to cases where the cancer originates primarily in the peritoneum rather than the ovaries.

The exact cause of peritoneal cancer is not well understood, but risk factors can include a family history of cancer and certain genetic mutations and a prior history of certain conditions or surgeries in the abdominal region.

The peritoneum and ovaries are two distinct structures in the abdominal region, but they are related in terms of their anatomical location and their involvement in certain diseases.

The peritoneum is a layer of tissue that lines the inner walls of the abdomen and pelvis. It covers and supports various abdominal organs, such as the stomach, liver, intestines, and reproductive organs like the uterus and fallopian tubes. The peritoneum acts as a protective barrier and also plays a role in the circulation and absorption of fluids within the abdominal cavity.

On the other hand, the ovaries are a pair of small, almond-shaped organs located on either side of the uterus in the female reproductive system. They are responsible for producing and releasing eggs (ova) during the menstrual cycle, as well as secreting hormones like estrogen and progesterone.

While the peritoneum covers and surrounds the pelvic structures, including the ovaries, peritoneal cancer specifically refers to cancer that originates primarily in the peritoneum rather than the ovaries. In contrast, ovarian cancer originates in the cells of the ovaries themselves.

Both peritoneal cancer and ovarian cancer can have similar symptoms, such as abdominal pain, bloating, and changes in bowel habits. They can also have similarities in terms of treatment approaches, often involving surgery and chemotherapy. However, the primary site of origin and the specific cells involved differentiate peritoneal cancer from ovarian cancer.

Treatment for peritoneal cancer typically involves a combination of surgery, chemotherapy, and occasionally radiation therapy. The specific treatment plan is tailored to the individual based on factors such as the stage of cancer, overall health, and preferences.

Early diagnosis and prompt treatment are important for better outcomes in peritoneal cancer. Regular medical check-ups, awareness of symptoms, and discussing any concerns with a healthcare provider can help in the early detection and management of peritoneal cancer.

Peritoneal cancer and epithelial cancer of the peritoneum are essentially the same thing. Epithelial cancer refers to cancer that originates in the cells that make up the epithelium, which is the outermost layer of cells in various organs and tissues, including the peritoneum.

Epithelial cancer of the peritoneum specifically refers to cancer that originates in the epithelial cells of the peritoneum. The peritoneum is a layer of tissue that lines the inner walls of the abdomen and covers the abdominal organs. It is composed of epithelial cells.

Peritoneal cancer can be further categorized into primary peritoneal cancer or secondary peritoneal cancer. Primary peritoneal cancer refers to cases where the cancer originates primarily in the peritoneum itself, while secondary peritoneal cancer occurs when cancer cells spread (metastasize) to the peritoneum from other primary sites, such as the ovaries, fallopian tubes, or gastrointestinal tract.

Epithelial cancer of the peritoneum, regardless of whether it is primary or secondary, presents with similar symptoms and is typically managed through surgery, chemotherapy, and other treatment modalities depending on the specific case and stage of the cancer.

It is essential to consult with a healthcare professional for an accurate diagnosis, personalized treatment plans, and proper management of epithelial cancer of the peritoneum.

This chapter specifically focuses on the treatment of epithelial cancer that develops in any of these three areas - ovarian, fallopian tube, and primary peritoneal cancer. They are closely related and treated in the same manner.

Harold Clinic

I enjoy sharing information about breathing issues related to diseases, such as lung cancer. These issues are similar in development and are related to other types of cancer.

I have put it through four stages to provide you with critical information for self-healing.

1.   Abdominal pain or irregularities
2.   Chest and sternum discomfort
3.   Nose issues
4.   Tonsil problems

As I take the stage, the primary root cause starts in the gut, just like other types of cancer do. This highlights my point that the lymphatic system is the first to be affected, from starting in the lymph to ending in the lymph, which is the hidden root of the defense system.

Cancer in the gut may begin as a small lump that moves around. As it becomes more solid, it may attach to blood vessels and grow larger. Eventually, it may protrude and feel firm to the touch. If you notice these symptoms, it is important to seek medical attention. The depth and severity of the cancer can vary depending on oxygen levels in the body. The virus may also spread from the gut to the chest and eventually to the tonsils, leading to the development of lung cancer.

Once you reach the moving stage, you may experience a slight pain in your arm or leg. This pain can affect the nerves or blood flow in that specific area, causing it to ache. This signals your brain to register the pain as described in the meridian theory, where the lung meridian passes through the inside of the arm. However, it is not considered serious at this stage. By the third or fourth stage, the pain becomes more intense and severe, often leading to various clinical cases involving leg, arm, or chest pain that can impact breathing.

Most cases involve the sternum, covering the heart and lungs, mostly in the middle of the chest area. This is caused by a virus, which affects the heart's irregular rhythm and causes shortness of breath when stress is present. This means that when your body is in fighting mode, the virus loves it because it causes your T cells or white blood cells to struggle. The virus is able to break free from your body's self-defense mechanisms, making it more active and causing you to feel even worse. Although you may not have an actual heart problem, you may feel as though you do because the virus is targeting the connecting point in the chest and sternum.

As mentioned in a previous discussion about skin topics, our bodies have various pathways that cross and intersect, moving up and down, as well as from right to left, connecting our internal organs to our skin. The vaccine acts like a reset or reboot for our body systems, though the visible effects are understood, the invisible consequences require further study and medical experimentation. We are not machines, but highly evolved human beings from millions of years ago.

The respiratory system, digestion, and lymphatic system all originate near the gut and are interconnected. Understanding these systems is crucial in a clinical setting as I point out that the lymphatic system is both the beginning and end. This is important because it directly relates to real cases experienced by many individuals.

As I explained in the three levels of disease affecting Eastern medicine, the first stage is the breathing skin level. Moving to the second stage, the muscles and tissues are affected. The final stage includes the blood level, organ level, or viscera level, which is a deeper level. Adding one more level, we refer to the bone level, which is reached in the last stage and represents the source of Jing essence. This is the final stage where the virus continues to spread more strongly and deeply, covering itself.

The virus steals your oxygen and pure blood to develop in the stage. The virus needs more oxygen and blood, making you feel more tired as you eat the same. Why is it so serious? You are in oxygen debt stage due to the virus. The more the virus takes your oxygen, the more it proliferates quickly, turning the stage where you either kill the virus or be killed by the virus.

The virus never goes away, building layers by stealing your oxygen. This is bad. The deeper layer and hardening tumor make it harder to treat, more sensitive, and lose momentum, accelerating quickly.

Why does the virus know when to turn the corner or gain momentum? They are waiting for you to make a mistake every day.

The treatment plan for your condition will be determined based on various factors, including the type, stage, and grade of your cancer, results from biomarker testing, the presence of an inherited mutation, the possibility of complete surgical removal of your tumor, and how your cancer reacts to treatment in Western medicine.

The number of previous treatments and therapies you have received (applicable for recurrent or advanced) will impact your treatment plan in the Eastern version. Check out chapter 2 of the Harold Clinic for more information.

In breast cancer, the virus infiltrates the dermal layer, forming a lump in the first stage. The worst part is that we often fail to recognize this viral invasion, allowing the tumor to grow and spread rapidly. This quick progression is due to the failure of the lymphatic defense in the armpit, providing the virus with an ideal environment to thrive with abundant food and soft tissue structure.

The first step is to check for any lumps or small tumors by screening or using your fingers regularly. Early detection is crucial, as small tumors can quickly spread and break down the lymphatic system. Treatment options may include surgery combined with chemotherapy or a three-dimensional approach using Eastern medicine techniques such as acupuncture, moxibustion, and magnet therapy outlined in chapter 2.

Root cause

I investigate the root causes of all chronic and COVID diseases. It is valuable to research in the modern medical community, taking into consideration both Western and Eastern medicine perspectives. Lastly, I draw my own conclusions based on clinical evidence and theoretical knowledge.

The intestine undergoes rapid turnover and regeneration to maintain its structural integrity and functionality. This constant renewal is crucial for preserving the barrier function of the gut, facilitating nutrient absorption, and protecting against pathogens and damage.

Your gut wall is designed to regenerate and flourish. These stem cells are exquisitely sensitive to vitamin D, which stimulates them to actively transform into gut wall cells. Adequate amounts of vitamin D (the form of D your body produces from sunlight on the skin, also available from some animal-sourced foods, and in supplement form) have a powerful ability to reverse fatigue. It certainly works wonders for my autoimmune patients, who are often deficient in this key nutrient. Could this be because vitamin D helps a leaky gut to heal, thus calming the inflammatory war inside?

At the base of each "root," known as villi, there exists a petite crypt that holds an extraordinary entity - intestinal stem cells. These stem cells play a crucial role in generating new cells for the lining of our gut in response to demand, alongside a repository of beneficial microbes.

A stem cell located in the crypt separates itself from its counterparts and ascends along the microvilli, akin to a crawl.

Taking a second perspective from the eastern medicine

The Sacral Chakra, located just below the navel, serves as the center of purification. Known as "Dantian," which translates to "field of elixir," this term refers to what many believe to be the reservoir of life force energy within the body. This concept originates from Taoist and Buddhist traditions and is thought to be connected to elevated states of consciousness. It connects to the liver (Lv), gallbladder (Gb), spleen (Sp), stomach (St), kidneys (Kd), bladder (Bl), intestines, skin, sexual orientation, and reproduction. It governs sexuality, creativity, and the development of relationships (getting along well with others). Mucosa-associated lymphoid tissue is located in gastrointestinal tract in the abdomen.

Initially, I discovered compelling evidence of "The Energy Paradox" by Steven R. Gundry, MD and "Drop Acid" by David Perlmutter with Kristin Loberg, MD. At the base of each villi, there is a small crypt that houses something very special - intestinal stem cells that aid in the production of new gut lining cells when needed, as well as a deposit of helpful microbes.

The description of the "root," or villi, as a small crypt containing intestinal stem cells that assist in the growth of new gut lining cells and helpful microbes, highlights an intriguing aspect of the structure and function of the intestine, particularly the small intestine. Let's delve into the significance of this statement:

Villi, which are finger-like projections found in the small intestine lining, increase the surface area available for nutrient absorption. They play a vital role in improving the efficiency of digestion and absorption of nutrients from food.

These specialized cells are located in the intestinal crypts, small pockets or invaginations in the intestine lining. Intestinal stem cells have the unique ability to divide and differentiate into different cell types, including those that form the gut lining.

The presence of intestinal stem cells in the crypts enables the continuous replenishment and repair of the gut lining. These cells can quickly multiply and change into new cells to replace damaged or worn-out ones, ensuring the integrity and functionality of the intestinal barrier.

In addition to intestinal stem cells, the crypts may also house a reservoir of beneficial microorganisms known as the gut microbiota. These microbes play a vital role in digestion, nutrient absorption, immune function, and overall gut health. Their presence in the crypts signifies the symbiotic relationship between the host and the microbiota.

Highlights the dynamic and complex nature of the intestinal environment, where stem cells, microbiota, and specialized structures like villi work together to maintain gut homeostasis, support nutrient absorption, and protect against infections and inflammation. The presence of intestinal stem cells within the crypts ensures the continuous renewal of the gut lining, while the coexistence of beneficial microbes contributes to overall gut health.

In embryology, Invagination is a key mechanism of morphogenesis, the biological process by which tissues and organs acquire their shape and structure. By folding inwards, cells create complex **three-dimensional structures** and compartments essential for the proper functioning of organs and systems within an organism.

At the cellular level, invagination can occur during processes such as gastrulation, where cells change shape and position to form **the three primary germ layers**—ectoderm, mesoderm, and endoderm. This inward folding of cells is critical for organizing cell populations and establishing tissue layers that will later differentiate into specific structures.

gut lining regenerates itself on a weekly basis and when a cell dies and needs to be replaced, a stem cell from the crypt literally divides itself from the others and "crawls" up the microvilli.

highlights the remarkable process of gut lining regeneration, which is a dynamic and essential function of the intestinal epithelium

The lining of the gastrointestinal tract, particularly the small intestine, undergoes rapid turnover and regeneration to maintain its structural integrity and functionality. This constant renewal is crucial for preserving the barrier function of the gut, facilitating nutrient absorption, and protecting against pathogens and damage.

Your gut wall is designed to regenerate and flourish. These stem cells are exquisitely sensitive to vitamin D, which stimulates them to actively transform to become a gut wall cell.so adequate amounts of vitamin D, (the form of D your body produces from sunlight on the skin, also available from some animal-sourced foods, and in supplement form) has an almost superpower to reverse fatigue, it certainly does wonders for my autoimmune patients, who are always deficient in this autoimmune improvement, general fatigue improvement could this be because vitamin Ds helps a leaky gut to heal, thus calming the inflammatory war inside

At the base of each "root," known as villi, exists a petite crypt that holds an extraordinary entity - intestinal stem cells. These stem cells play a crucial role in generating new cells for the lining of our gut in response to demand, alongside a repository of beneficial microbes.

a stem cell located in the crypt separates itself from its counterparts and ascend along the microvilli, akin to a crawl.

Root cause of the lymphatic point of view

Mucosa-associated lymphoid tissue is located in the subclavian vein.

The mesenteric lymph nodes are responsible for draining the gastrointestinal tract in the abdomen, and they are a part of the gastrointestinal-associated lymphoid tissue (GALT).

In conclusion, the small intestine produces the main lymph fluids, known as chyle, in the gut. The large intestine then circulates lymph fluid to detox in the gut.

When it comes to viruses, the large intestine plays a significant role in detoxifying the gut. I believe the root cause lies first in the large intestine and second in the small intestine, which produces the lymph fluids.

I agree that lymph fluids are the root cause, but there is some disagreement on which organ is primarily responsible. Based on the principle of oxygen awareness and blood flow, the large intestine lymph is aware that viruses are not being invaded.

The large intestine is a yang organ, followed by the lung as the yin paring organ. Therefore, I believe that all root causes lie in the large intestine, with colon cancer being the primary concern and lung cancer being secondary due to the yin organ being more severe than the yang organ, which just plays a role in making it empty but yin is more related to blood, causing more damage to occur.

According to the meridian theory, the small intestine meridian circulates to the neck, along the same line as the clavicle lymphatic line to the ear. Similarly, the large intestine meridian also circulates to the neck, along the same line as the clavicle lymphatic line to the nose.

Combining both Eastern and Western medicine, Eastern medicine suggests that the main producer of chyle in the small intestine is circulated to the neck by the meridian theory, all connected to protect against virus invasion of the brain. The lymphatic system in the neck plays a crucial role in fighting off viruses and chronic diseases.

When it comes to detoxing, many people associate it with the liver, but in reality, only blood is processed there. Lymph does not travel to the liver; instead, it goes straight to the lungs to defend against invisible air. The detoxing process is not visible - blood is created in the spleen with earthy energy, and lymph fluid works with oxygen, which is qi or heavenly energy. The detoxing process actually begins in the large intestine through the Lymphatic system, which is the true root cause. Lung disease can result from a defect in the lymph function of the large intestine.

Anthony William has a negative opinion of blood tests, which I agree with. This is because not all viruses and lymph fluids are located in the blood vessels; some are in the dynamic movement of fighting invisible lymph fluids within the skin layer. As a result, it is probable that many COVID and chronic patients have a deficiency in their blood. The more blood tests that are conducted, the greater the likelihood of identifying these deficiencies.

Case study

Kevin, who is in his 60s, has been dealing with breathing and digestion issues for a long time. He has suffered from chronic runny nose and took pills when he was young. When he started a stressful job at 30, he began experiencing chest pain and a fear of breathing problems. Additionally, he started to experience brain fog and had difficulty completing tasks. Throughout his life, he has struggled with chronic tiredness and low energy, accepting it as his genetic predisposition. Feeling like he has lost his potential, he is now exploring Eastern medicine for answers. He realized the connection between his digestive and breathing issues, both centered around his belly. It was a long journey to find a treatment that worked for him.

The primary issue with breathing often lies in chest-related heart palpitations, alongside symptoms like tonsillitis and nasal congestion. The root cause of these problems is not located in the lungs, but rather in the gut, where there is a tumor present.

At the clinic, we observe that toxic buildup first occurs in the gut, not the lungs or in the nasal passages. This can be explained by understanding the basic functions of the lymphatic system, which is linked to the small intestine and circulates through the large intestine.

According to the principles of Yin and Yang, an imbalance occurs when Yang energy initiates movement and Yin energy subsequently responds, similar to how oxygen and blood circulate. Therefore, addressing these issues involves focusing on the following:

1. Respiratory health,
2. Digestive processes, particularly lymphatic function,
3. The condition of the gut, especially near lymphatic tissues.

The Third Eye Chakra with lymphatic system

Anus breathing

Upper position indang Brain, nasal breathing in brain

Middle position – danjung Heart, moderate thoracic breathing in the
heart

Lower position – gwanwon Abdomen, abdominal breathing in the gut

Rem sleep and lymphatic flow

Master said eastern medicine have not clear concept of brain

Why eastern any anatomy of brain why take it seriously why

And why hormone is critical most western medicine why not in
eastern medicine

Why is that

Why no deep research no make sense

That is true but no surgery just many option of treatment by needle
or heat or magnet

In the clinic, there are more options available than just applying
stimuli and improving circulation, as compared to Western medicine.

The brain is composed of the cerebral hemisphere, cerebellum,
and brainstem. The surface is made up of gray matter, while the inner
part consists of white matter. The cortex is responsible for all mental
activities.

In Western medicine, there is a wealth of information available on
the brain. It is said that, on average, the brain uses 20% of the body's
total energy expenditure during certain cognitive tasks or periods of
high mental activity, increasing to around 25-40%.

We see things differently when it comes to the brain. In Eastern medicine, there is no concept of the brain having three organs and six meridians passing through it. Unlike Western medicine, Eastern medicine focuses on cosmic principles.

The brain is a complex organ composed of five organs assembled together. Each organ has its own function, and when combined, they create a more complex function. The brain is essential, just like the other five organs

The brainstem is connected to the heart, liver, and spleen. The midbrain is connected to the heart and liver. The cerebellum is connected to the gallbladder and triple burner. The pituitary gland is connected to the heart, kidney, and liver. The spinal cord performs its function by connecting the liver and kidney, playing a central role in coordinating reflex movements.

There are a total of nine openings in the body: the mouth, nose, front yin penis, anus, eyes (2), and ears (2). The body is composed of five elements: skin, muscle, bone, flesh, and hair.

Five emotions - anger, joy, worry, thinking, and sadness - are connected to the five senses: sight, hearing, smell, taste, and touch. This linkage explains the relationship between the five organs and the principles of cosmic change within the human body. The theory of the five organ meridians is a fundamental concept in clinical verification and Understanding 5 organ 6 bu studies is crucial for effective clinical practice.

Sleep is essential because during this time, our bodies connect to invisible energy and the lymphatic system kicks in to detoxify and purify our blood and body fluids. Sleeping allows our bodies to reboot and repair. Different people have various sleep patterns, and improper sleep can lead to health issues such as insufficient oxygen for erectile tissue and a build-up of toxins in the body. The quality of sleep can reveal the true functioning of the body, with factors like breathing patterns impacting sleep quality.

For example, if you are experiencing breathing issues, check the circadian time from 3 am to 5am . Additionally, ensure your nose is properly breathing; otherwise, your sleep quality may be low. Check whether both nostrils are clear or not. Many people are only able to breathe through one nostril, meaning they are only utilizing 50% of their breathing capacity. If both nostrils are not clear, resorting to mouth breathing is not ideal, as it can have negative effects on your immune system. Without proper oxygen and mucus, the air you breathe in can become toxic.

It is the primary cause of chronic respiratory diseases. To learn how to treat it, refer to chapter 2.

Sleep supports the brain's own detoxification system, known as the glymphatic system, which cleans up metabolic waste and toxins that build up throughout the day. Our daily biological rhythms are influenced by our exposure to light: sunlight in the morning and darkness at night.

Brain waves transition from hype beta waves to calming alpha waves, and eventually to low delta waves during deep sleep. In this state, the brain is composed of swirling atomic particles - it is energy, it is prana.

From a Western perspective, the ventricles in the brain are chambers filled with cerebrospinal fluid (CSF). Each cerebral hemisphere contains a lateral ventricle. CSF is produced by the choroid plexus and circulates through the ventricles and spinal cord canal. It then enters the subarachnoid space through openings and flows through the subarachnoid space of the brain and spinal cord. CSF is absorbed by the arachnoid villi and returned to the venous system. If the reabsorption of CSF is blocked in infancy, hydrocephalus, also known as "water on the brain," can develop, causing the ventricles to enlarge and the cortex to thin.

The brain receives a constant amount of blood flow, around 20% at rest which decreases during exercise but the total flow increases. There is little difference in blood flow between rest and exercise.

The brain has a high metabolism and uses glucose for energy, requiring a constant supply of glucose. It also has a high demand for oxygen - interruption of oxygen supply can lead to rapid neuron death.

A clinical condition known as strokes, or cerebrovascular accidents (CVA), can occur.

Interrupting blood supply to the brain typically involves a large artery. A stroke can be caused by three different mechanisms: thrombosis, embolism, and hemorrhage. Thrombosis occurs when a blood vessel narrows, leading to complete blockage (known as a thrombus) that cuts off blood supply to the rest of the artery and surrounding brain tissue. This accounts for over 50% of all strokes. Embolism occurs when a material such as a blood clot, fat body, or bacterial clump travels from another part of the body and becomes lodged in a narrowing vessel. This type of stroke accounts for less than 20% of cases. Hemorrhage, the least common type of stroke, involves the rupture of a blood vessel, releasing blood into the surrounding tissue. Not only is blood supply cut off, but the escaping blood also acts as a foreign object occupying space. Hemorrhages account for less than 20% of strokes but are often fatal.

Hariold Clinic

Eastern medicine emphasizes the importance of the Du-20 Baihui acupoint, also known as the Hundred Meetings point, in achieving optimal brain blood circulation. It is recommended to use small Japanese moxa to stimulate this point, This point is considered miraculous for the brain as it has the ability to reduce brain heat, expand vessels for a hypo brain, and lower high blood pressure by expelling heat. Both of these functions are readily available.

Respected researchers, such as Dr. Jonathan Kipnis of the University of Virginia and Dr. Maiken Nedergaard who studied the role of lymph in the brain, have made important discoveries in the field. While it was previously believed that the central nervous system did not contain the lymphatic system, Dr. Kipnis and his team found markers for lymphatics in vessels in mice.

Upon further examination, it was discovered that lymphatic tissue is linked to the glymphatic system as a way to remove toxins from the brain. This process involves drainage through the nasal mucosa and lymphatics of the cranial nerves. The lymph is responsible for draining waste, including beta-amyloid, via cerebral spinal fluid to large veins. This process is most active during the rapid eye movement (REM) cycle of sleep, occurring in 15- to 30-minute cycles per night. During this time, about 70 percent of the clearance of amyloid plaques takes place.

Research indicates that sleeping on your side, rather than on your back, is associated with better clearance. However, the system does not always function effectively, possibly due to inadequate lymphatic circulation. It is important to practice methods to improve lymphatic flow to enhance this process and prevent a buildup of toxins.

Studies have shown that patients with Alzheimer's disease have accumulations of debris in their cerebral-spinal fluid, highlighting the significance of clearing this debris. The lymph plays a crucial role in clearing debris, transporting it through the lymph nodes and lymph paths to the liver for metabolism and elimination. Early research suggests that the lymph is essential for keeping the brain free of substances that can obstruct neural connections. This cleansing process is crucial not only in Alzheimer's disease but also in other neurological disorders like Parkinson's disease.

Harold Clinic

the secret technique of transforming stupidity into genius known as the masking technique. The key factor in determining the quality of blood flow to the brain is the carotid artery. It is widely accepted in academic circles that Albert Einstein's intelligence did not surpass that of others due to his brain alone, but rather because his neuronal glial cells and blood flow through his carotid artery were consistently superior.

An effective and simple way to improve blood flow in the carotid artery is by holding a paper bag over the mouth and taking deep breaths for 30 seconds. It is recommended for children to do this under the supervision of adults. While CO_2 therapy is available in large hospitals with advanced machines, it can be costly for each session. Therefore, it is advised to perform the masking therapy every 30 minutes, especially during breaks from work or school.

Regular practice of the masking technique can enhance cerebral circulation, improve the brain's nutritional status, strengthen blood vessels, and boost cognitive functions such as thinking, senses, memory, understanding, and emotions. It may also help in preventing strokes. Combining natural foods with this technique can lead to optimal results.

CO_2 therapy and the masking technique have the same meaning: holding your breath. This triggers the counteractive production of oxygen in our body, which is have the same effect of stimulating the body to produce the oxygen it needs. This process counteracts the body's natural mechanisms.

I recommend practicing anus breathing. I do it every morning from 3 am to 7am . Start by inhaling and being aware of the air flowing smoothly into the brain, neck, and lungs. Next, gently close the anus and hold your breath for as long as you can. Count slowly from 1 to 10, then 20, 30, 50, and finally 100 before exhaling.

As you hold your breath longer, your heart begins to pound and your body temperature slowly rises, causing more blood to circulate in your toxic areas. I feel a vibration in my pinky finger, signaling that my heart meridian is activated, which is amazing. This is the best time for natural and effective results.

Start your day with a daily detox routine to clear away inner debris, which is indicated by yawning and watery eyes, as it signifies the release of toxic gases and fluids from your body - a positive detoxification sign. Follow this up by detoxing for the new day, bringing in more oxygen to clear your brain and generate new ideas. As new energy is produced and waste is eliminated, you may begin to feel hungry, so be sure to eat plenty of fruits, milk, and protein. Embrace the wonderful new morning, as it marks the start of a heavenly natural detox hour.

Detoxify Your Body Naturally with Heavenly Hour Detox

There are times when I treat myself by waking up naturally at 3 am after going to bed before 10 pm, which is considered the best time for detox. During the first REM sleep cycle, the lymph fluid is released, and the body begins to heal itself, stretching with new energy. REM sleep is the optimal time to dream and connect to healing energy, allowing your body to relax and avoid wasting energy.

Clearing your nose and breathing in oxygen during this time feels like a heavenly massage in your dreams, leading to new ideas and decisions. Many successful people follow this routine, and I am grateful for the oxygen treatment and the new thoughts it has brought me. Remember to consider the circadian hour for your daily rituals.

From 11 pm to 1 am, the gallbladder releases bile, repairs cells, and builds blood. From 1 am to 3 am, it is the liver's detox time for blood cleansing. Then, from 3 am to 5 am, the detox process begins with universal energy entering your lungs.

From 11pm to 3am, the body detoxifies all waste from the previous day. From 3am to 5am, it begins to generate new energy for the new day. This process occurs in a sequence. If it is not properly activated, you may feel tired even after a long sleep. Therefore, it is important to feel energized after sleeping, whether it is for a short or long period of time. Maintaining a regular sleep pattern is crucial for obtaining the best energy levels.

Between 5am and 7am, it is important to awaken the large intestine by promoting lymphatic vessel movement for detoxification purposes.

This time is ideal for engaging in activities such as meditation, attending a yoga class, or participating in prayer at a church or temple. This is when heavenly energy naturally descends, providing us with the best air quality and nature's breath that our bodies need.

Chapter 2

Self-Treatment

YAMM Treatment

It is time to consider Eastern medicine treatments option instead of relying solely on surgery and chemotherapy. Having a compromised immune system will provide you with more treatment options for both COVID patients and patients with chronic diseases. I refer to it as the YAMM treatment., incorporates Yoga breathing, Acupuncture, Moxibustion, and Magnet treatment, all without any side effects.

Acupuncture helps in connecting the body's electrolytes, moxibustion uses heat to break down toxic proteins and thick calcification tissue, and magnet treatment assists in balancing the body fluids' pH levels. By combining these three techniques, we can effectively combat various chronic diseases by disrupting the virus's communication, breaking down virus colonies, and detoxifying the body fluids naturally. This approach aims to recover and heal the lymph fluids in a natural and efficient way.

Chronic Disease Case Treatment: A Case Study

This case involves a general chronic condition in a woman over the age of 60. She experiences a variety of mixed symptoms, including pain that is scattered throughout her body, making it difficult to pinpoint the root cause.

After a thorough examination, the primary concerns identified were related to her respiratory system as the first issue and the gut, specifically the small intestine, as the second. Additionally, we need to address the large intestine for internal detoxification, as described in Chapter 1.

1. **How to treat collaborated with Eastern medicine and Western Medicine?**
2. **General symptoms of after age 58 urinary tract infection with Kidney issue**
3. **Emotional pain causing adrenaline surge with mood swings more instant sugar craving**

Here is her own word

The first reason I came to clinic was for sugar addition and my bladder incontinence Then I thought that I wasn't getting my back loosened up with the chiropractor so I thought I should try acupuncture for that as well

I have a hectic day and I feel that I can rewind at night with a movie, glass of wine and comfort food. I have been doing this on a constant basis since my daughter passed away.

She was all I had and my whole life. If you have any other guesting feel free to text me

Patient medications:
1. Veniafaxine HCL XR-375mg (once daily)
2. Clonazepam -0.25mg (3 daily)
3. Lamotrigine – 25 mg (3 tablets twice daily)

4. Zopiclone - -7.5 mg (once daily)
Consider Medication drawback affecting Kidney

Patient Supplement
Vitamine B Complex,C D3,E
Salmon Oil, Magnesium Citrate
Glucosamine, Chondroitin, and MSM

Lysine Calcium Osteo Joint Ease (with Glucosamine, Chondroitin, and MSM)

Patient's Diet:**
- **Breakfast:** Steel-cut oats with blueberries, flaxseed, and applesauce.
- **Lunch:** Sandwich or salad. **Dinner:** Chicken with vegetables, pizza, or pasta.
- **Daytime Snacks:** Apple, banana, cucumber, carrots.
- **Evening Snacks:** A glass of wine with cheese and crackers

Patient's Condition:
- A uric acid level of **2.19 umol/L** is considered low, as it falls below the normal reference range of **150-360 umol/L
*A high-normal level does not rule out gout.
Magnesium Level: 360 um (or **750 to 950 μmol/L**).
- **Glucose Level (AC):** 5.1 mmol/L (Normal range: 3.8-6.0 AC = Ante Cibum)
- **Hemoglobin A1c:** 4.8 to 5.4% normal
- **Fasting Blood Glucose:** <95 mg/dL normal
- **Fasting Insulin:** <8 IU/mL (Ideally <3 IU/mL) insuline resistance

Assessment Plan:

1. Begin by examining her back.
2. Next, assess her breathing.
3. Address bladder inconsistency, which may indicate detoxification issues.

The patient frequently reports elbow pain, which appears straightforward. However, the root cause seems to be toxic buildup both physically and emotionally throughout her life. The back exhibits significant tightness and stiffness, especially in the upper and middle thoracic regions (T3 to T7). Some of the lactic acid is present as sodium lactate in the blood, is

excreted through the kidneys. The majority is burned or reconverted into glycogen. This burning process occurs after exercise has ceased.

Therefore, we are able to continue working beyond the limits set by the available oxygen, but only if we later intake enough oxygen to burn off the accumulated waste. This results in what has been referred to as an "oxygen debt

Meaning middle Jio Liver and Gut function is not normal

Second her breathing close one nostil the other she got a tonsil surgery long time ago
Meaning her tonsil auto nerve system not working
Tonsil infection curable but it surgery to cut it out no chance to get nerve back meaning
Detox breathing job failed empty breathing cause some panic case
First acupuncture at indang point small dose of toxic blood out she is happy to breathing better

About tonsilitis

Many case in that expecially kids kids

Take, for example, the time when tonsillectomies first drew favor. Many children began presenting with tonsillitis, and the prevailing wisdom became that the tonsils should be removed. It became such dominant thinking that no one even thought to question whether the cause of tonsillitis in the first place could be addressed instead. The focus on the medical advancement of the tonsillectomy procedure completely buried the mystery of this widespread tonsillitis. Once tonsillectomies became commonplace, someone in medical school wouldn't be encouraged to probe the problem anymore, because it had become "been there, done that" Remove the tonsils, the thinking went, and remove the problem. Why spend any more time thinking about it?

Medical communities now recognize that the tonsils are tied into the immune system, and so removing them isn't the best first option when they're infected. Now antibiotics have become the favored first line of defense. This is problem-atic, because while cofactor bacteria can further inflame the tonsils, bacteria are not the underlying cause of tonsillitis; EBV is. This whole time, it's been juvenile Epstein-Barr virus causing inflamed tonsils. In children, EBV is very difficult to diagnose, because it often doesn't raise red flags that testing can detect in the bloodstream.

Meanwhile, the lymphatic area where the tonsils reside can become infected as they try to fight off the virus, causing the mystery tonsil infection. It's another instance of hidden mono-nucleosis-and the history of medical research and science being mistaken about how to solve a problem.

**Initial Assessment of Treatment: **

Gut and Respiratory Conditions: First Evaluation
- Uric Acid: Low pH levels indicate an acidic gut, increasing vulnerability to infections.
- Liver Function: Operating at approximately half capacity.
- Brain Health: Patient is taking a pill to aid sleep.
- Emotional Impact: Depletion of glucose in the brain due to emotional stress.
- Adrenaline Response: The body is activating the adrenaline hormone for emergency responses, leading to increased cravings for sugar.
- Glucose Levels: There is a lack of glucose reserves in both the brain and liver, contributing to insulin resistance. Possible factors include low magnesium levels, dietary animal fats, or viral infections.
- Vital Signs: The patient's pulse is notably weak, indicating that blood and oxygen levels are significantly below normal.

In summary, this complex, chronic condition appears to stem from inadequate oxygen supply.

Breathing exercises should be prioritized first, followed by gut recovery, with a focus on slow and steady long-term treatment.

The positive aspect is that she has secured a job, which means daily movement is beneficial for her health.

Her conditions appear to be the result of a combination of physical and mental toxicity, viewed from an Eastern perspective. At 58 years of age, there is a notable depletion of Kidney Yang and Liver Spleen Qi, along with blood deficiency, which are potential root causes of her depression, anxiety, and insomnia.

From a diagnostic standpoint, pulse and tongue assessments indicate blood deficiency and a low energy level. There is significant stiffness in both sides of the thoracic muscles, particularly from T3 to T7, suggesting almost complete dysfunction of the associated nerves and muscles. It is advisable to first examine the spinal cord and the immune system, utilizing acupuncture at the Indang point.

For breathing difficulties, liver supplements and nasal acupuncture can be beneficial. Additionally, Japanese tiny moxibustion should be performed on the T3 to T7 vertebrae during each clinic visit.

Detoxifying liver supplements can raise the body's temperature using medical heat lamps, moxibustion, and hot tub baths.

In terms of diet, incorporating celery juice and fruits with natural sugars, such as blueberries,pear, and grapes, is recommended. To help address bladder incontinence, include cauliflower, broccoli, and green vegetables to combat insulin resistance.

Healing will take time, with approximately 30 clinic sessions required. The treatment program will aim to:

1. Boost the immune system with acupuncture at the nose.
2. Improve the body's metabolism through the use of heat lamps and Japanese tiny moxibustion, or using stick moxa on the tense muscles at the back.
3. Address urinary infections and bladder inconsistencies.

For most women over the age of 58, health issues can become more complex. A history of C-sections and gallbladder surgery can leave behind toxins in the body, creating an environment conducive to the Strep virus.

For treatment, acupuncture combined with Japanese moxibustion at the Kidney point can help eliminate this virus.

What lies at the root of these issues? The underlying cause often stems from the gut and respiratory system. Women frequently experience a deficiency pattern characterized by coldness, lack of warmth, and depression. Issues such as thyroid failure and leaky gut can adversely affect brain function via the vagus nerve.

In Eastern medicine, we have a plan B treatment option based on whether a patient exhibits excess (hyper) or deficient (hypo) symptoms:

- For excess types: Acupuncture, bloodletting, cupping therapy,
- For deficient types: Japanese tiny moxibustion, acupressure, herbal supplements, and massage are recommended.

After undergoing a significant life event, many women tend to shift to a deficient state, which can be confirmed by weak pulses. In cases of excess, the first step is to check for a strong pulse. For example, one patient's sister visited me after being referred; her condition was distinctly different.

Interestingly, her older sister is an excess type. She was born with strong genetic traits, which is evident in her robust and healthy pulse. However, she has expressed concerns about her sleep.

In her 20s, she experienced shingles, which presented as a small patch on her side during exam time, but medication successfully cleared it up. She has three grown children, all delivered naturally. At 45, she underwent a tubal ligation and had one other surgical procedure to remove excess tissue from under her armpit.

As an excess type, the key for her is to reduce heat. I inquired if she consumes animal products.

Oxygen: No surplus, only debt

Oxygen is never in surplus; it is always in demand, influencing us every second. However, we often take for granted the air we breathe. How much oxygen do we truly receive? It's likely less than we think, especially when considering the impact of infections.

To put it simply, without oxygen, one can only survive for about four minutes before succumbing to death. Many severe health issues like stroke result from a lack of oxygen levels, highlighting the importance of ensuring adequate oxygen intake into the lungs.

Chronic diseases and prolonged COVID-19 are directly associated with oxygen debt, which is a central theme of my book. The fundamental functions of metabolism and energy production in the body are closely linked to oxygen, making it even more crucial than the lymphatic system.

Let us explore the role of oxygen in detail.

A new study reveals that the metabolic process of phosphorylation is responsible for transmitting signals related to oxygen levels in the blood and between cells. In the absence of oxygen, the body produces only 2 ATP, while the presence of oxygen allows for the production of 33 to 36 ATP. This means that when oxygen is available, ATP production can be up to 15 times more efficient. It's well-known among many that sufficient oxygen in the blood can lead to the generation of 33 to 36 ATP, whereas a lack of oxygen results in only 2 ATP.

The ability of muscles to take in oxygen and carry out the reverse processes is a remarkable feature. Oinuma demonstrated that an increase in carbon dioxide and temperature accelerates the release of oxygen. When muscles contract repeatedly, they generate not only additional carbon dioxide but also extra heat. These new conditions facilitate a more rapid and thorough release of oxygen from its carriers. Even during moderate exercise, the rate of oxygen liberation can double due to the influence of carbon dioxide, compounded by the rise in temperature within the active muscles. Simultaneously, the cells consume oxygen more quickly, resulting in a decrease in the oxygen levels within the lymph that surrounds them. This creates a steeper diffusion gradient from the blood to the lymph, leading to faster diffusion.

This is a key concept of the book: Why do we hold our breath, and why do breath-holding exercises last for 5, 10, 20, 50, or even 100 seconds?

This practice generates a comparable amount of oxygen. That is why we use masks to create an antagonistic effect—restricting oxygen intake and increasing carbon dioxide levels. Ultimately, this process helps to produce an equivalent amount of oxygen that diffuses into the lymphatic system.

The magic of breathing lies in the power of oxygen. Additionally, engaging in physical exercise while breathing properly can generate up to 30 times more ATP than what is typically possible for everyone.

It is important to note that these relationships are interconnected; as muscular activity increases, the effects on the rate of oxygen dissociation from the blood corpuscles and its movement to the cells also intensify. Therefore, the advantages of enhanced blood flow through the muscle capillaries are efficiently utilized.

The more rapid the separation of oxygen the higher will be its diffusion pressure in the plasma, and therefore, in turn, the more quickly will it pass into the lymph and thence into the active cells.

One notable mechanism for ensuring an adequate supply of oxygen during times of need is the rapid increase in red blood cell count that occurs during muscular exercise. This phenomenon, which Barcroft has notably clarified, is more pronounced in lower animals than in humans. For example, in horses, the number of red blood cells per cubic millimeter can rise by as much as 20 percent or more as a result of just five minutes of intense activity. This remarkable adaptation is the sole physiological response to oxygen deficit that resembles the storage mechanisms I have previously described in the context of homeostasis for other essential supplies.

During severe and prolonged muscular exertion, glucose is mobilized from liver reserves and distributed via the bloodstream to tissues that require it. When discussing the body's response to hemorrhage, it is important to note the spleen, which acts as a reservoir for red blood cells. Under conditions that stimulate the sympathico-adrenal system—such as those that prompt increased oxygen demand—the muscles of the spleen contract and release concentrated red blood cells into circulation. In cats, for instance, exercise may lead to a reduction in spleen weight from 26 grams to 13 grams, resulting in the release of 13 grams of fluid that is especially rich in red blood cells. These cells immediately function as carriers of oxygen and carbon dioxide, becoming essential when their services are most needed.

The complexity of these various mechanisms for maintaining homeostasis in oxygen delivery to the organism's fixed and secluded cells underscores the critical importance of continually adjusting this delivery to meet physiological demands.

Low-oxygen states can accelerate aging, a phenomenon often associated with obstructive sleep apnea. These conditions impact the body similarly to stress by triggering changes in the function of sirtuins, AMP-activated protein kinase (AMPK), and mTOR. They also reduce inflammation and enhance insulin sensitivity. Additionally, low-oxygen environments promote the production of stem cells and the formation of new blood vessels, allowing the body to acquire more oxygen.

While it may be impractical to climb to 10,000 feet every day, there are now devices that can simulate both low- and high-oxygen states. These devices replicate the experience of ascending Mount Everest for a few minutes, then descending to sea level or even a higher oxygen environment. This intermittent hypoxia-hyperoxia appears to induce numerous beneficial effects, including improved blood sugar control and cognitive function in dementia patients, as well as enhanced overall mitochondrial health. Low-oxygen states can lead to the elimination of older mitochondria while stimulating the formation of new, healthier ones—all essential for maintaining energy and promoting longevity.

It is more complicated for most women after age 58. history of C-session and gallbladder surgery left toxins to the habitat of the Strep virus

Acupuncture with Japan tiny Moxibustion at Kidney for kill off the virus

What is the root cause?

Again root cause in the gut and breathing Women deficiency pattern getting cold, no heat and depression

Thyroid failure and Leaky Gut affecting brain function by vagus verve

Eastern medicine plan b treatment option

Excess (hyper)type: Acupuncture, Bloodletting, Cupping Therapy
              Herb and Supplement and Massage
   Deficient (hypo) type: Japan Tiny Moxibustion, Acupressure
              Herb and Supplement and Massage

But most case woman after mana pose go to deficient type confirming by her pulse weak

Who is excess first check the pulse is strong Her sister visit me next day refer to me

So different

Interesting her old sister is excess type first she was bone to strong gene her pulse is strong and health

But her complain is sleep

She had a singles when 20 at exam time it was a small patch in my side and the meds cleared it up I have 3 children all grown all natural births had a tubular when I was 45 the only other surgery was an extraction of excess tissue under the my arm pit tube tied to prevent pregnancy

She is an excess type just reduce the heat I ask her do you animal meat no more she said no that is okay why after age 60 we need more protein for muscle and tissue than when young But she is not enough protein go to sugar addiction so different

Why gene and environment

I treated 25 times it cover daily detox but not root cause

She hate to moxa cus pain

That is a little different e and w by pain respond see the pain chapter

Gut see her diet she eat good nutrition but eat and absorb in gut is not same

Absorbing small intestine is normal she have a sugar addiction all eat and drink maybe half of it not absorbed it wasted see the bladder inconsistency is the pelvic floor or anus rectum function is below the normal meaning detox and oxygen intake problem show that

The first thing to do is detox and Gut function restore

Detox come from the supplement of liver detox to increase the liver function.

celery juice for gut restore to absorb the nutrition.

Indang point placed in between eye acupuncture

to inhale more oxygen

magnesium is the synthesize of the nutrition for cell tissue that need it need more than before

Glucose level the thing is glucose in the brain and liver reserve not enough daily activity.

But she all used up by emotional pain so need quick glucose leading sugar addition.

To prevent of insulin resistance, get the sugar from fruits

important sugar in fruits quick absorbing into cell within one hour but she need more energy first quick pizza

Grief causes qi to become stagnated and consumed Prolonged sorrow results in depression, which consumes lung qi

Yoga breathing

I see young girls with yoga mat in shoulder in the morning go to the class remind me of hot yoga in Vancouver that I did it lots of sweat why all circulation with heat that need to the cold aversion type of constitution called metal or type 2 personality

I did another type of breathing meditation 30 years ago the same like young guys at that time can not breath the way teaching just relax and short sleep is enough I think do not know the deep meaning of oxygen breathing that I do it every morning now

The less oxygen virus use your oxygen gain the strength feel more pain

So until kill the virus you have to be through the pain it natural so by breathing more effective the treatment most breathing is not consider your body condition now time to consider that and learn the breathing correctly know the principle apply it

Some level 2 stage some level 3 more deeper level more right breathing with treatment combined called healing breaching first check the your chest in the stunum core location of virus hinder your oxygen breathing

Why hold breath creating co2 purposely to increase the oxygen paradox it true

I feel it everyday why it heal everything holding breath counting 20 30 40 50 60 closing the anus rectum that is the same function of lung together more dynamic why it tang and yin breathing

This connection between blood pH and respiration rate is important for maintaining homeostasis in the body. Carbon dioxide levels affect the pH of the blood, and the respiratory system plays a vital role in regulating these levels. When the blood becomes too acidic, the respiratory system increases respiration rate to remove excess CO_2 and increase blood pH. On the other hand, when the blood becomes too alkaline, the respiratory system decreases respiration rate to retain CO_2 and lower blo

on Buteyko Breathing Education is a measurement called the control pause, which involves timing how long you can comfortably hold

your breath following an exhalation.

According to the Buteyko Clinic International, having a control pause of less than 25 seconds is considered poor, and 25 to 35 seconds means there's room for improvement.

The goal is to reach a comfortable breath-hold time of 40 or more seconds. The average control pause of students attending Buteyko clinics worldwide is around 15 seconds.

Students attend to help improve their asthma, dysfunctional breathing, anxiety, and sleep problems. With each five-second improvement to their control pause, breathing becomes lighter and the student feels better.

Eastern and harold breathing education is a little different than Buteyko Clinic

Breathing in first and hold it

Why Buteyko Clinic is for hyper ventilation type of person like Buteyko himself that he had a high blood pressure, so it is okay, contracting of blood vessel first of breathing

But most lung breathing issue person struggling hypo ventilation expanding blood vessel first and release

Again Adam 1 type of person, heat type of person, wood and fire elementary type person going to breath out first for contracting

Adam 2 type of person like hypo aversion to cold type of person, metal and water elementary person prone to contracting blood vessel going to breath in first for expanding

This is why using drugs to suppress symptoms can be so risky.

While they may provide temporary relief and improved functionality, the underlying disease processes continue to progress rapidly and our clues for treatments become obscured. Even worse, symptom-suppressing drugs delay the start of curative treatment.

suppress symptoms meaning making symptom contracting and narrowing for lung patients

As a result, recovery becomes longer and more challenging - more challenging because delaying the start of treatment runs the risk of additional complications arising. To overcome this terrible illness, one must take on the role of their own doctor.

The purpose of this book is to provide you with the guidelines and tools necessary to achieve this. This includes becoming knowledgeable about your symptoms and how you respond to treatments so that you can determine the root cause of the issue, why it's happening, and most importantly, how to implement a cure. Self-awareness is the foundation of true wisdom.

New study shows that the metabolic process of phosphorylation that transmits signal to blood by oxygen between cell
If not oxygen just 2 ATP if oxygen available 33 to 36 ATP possible

Meaning how to created the atp 15 times more power energy produce
It is most old people to know that
So oxygen in blood perfectly it goes 33 to 36 atp
Just no clear oxygen just 2 atp

Western breathing is confined to Obstruction Syndrome or restricted lung disease
As we see Obstructing and restricting means simply contraction, narrowing just for need expansion by heat or oxygen breathing

Harold clinic

Most infection start in it here located in the center of the breastbone,
at the fourth intercostal space (space between ribs), which is usually at the level of the nipples in men
virus starting it this and moving up to the face or brain

the same it form the thoracic duct
THORACIC DUCT: This is the body's largest lymphatic vessel, originating in the abdomen and running along the center of the body. It returns lymphatic fluid to the bloodstream near the neck at the left subclavian vein.

Eastern medicine refers to the Conception line, which is situated in the middle of the body and contains all the chakra points. Imagine if we were to divide our body straight down the middle into right and left sides from the lips to the penis, how would that look? I said that the left side represents blood and the right side represents energy. It is the connection point that becomes vulnerable when the virus invades.
There are two primary meridians in Eastern medicine known as

the Conception Channel and the Governor Channel, which serve as the main points for diagnosis and treatment.

When symptoms become severe, diseases typically start in the Conception channel where the chakras are located.

The Sacral Chakra, located below the navel, is a place of purification. It is connected to various organs and systems in the body and governs aspects such as sexuality, creativity, and relationships with others

Put it this on western version The mesenteric lymph nodes, responsible for draining the gastrointestinal tract in the abdomen, are located in this area. They are part of the gastrointestinal-associated lymphoid tissue (GALT).

In contrast, the channel in the governor vessel runs along the center of the back and initially receives signals from the atmosphere through the spinal cord. One pathway runs from the upper lip to the anus, generating positive electricity, while the other runs from the lower lip to the inside of the anus, producing negative energy. Therefore, it is essential to keep the lips sealed to facilitate electrical connection. This is why it is crucial to avoid mouth breathing and instead focus on breathing through the anus to activate energy.

Natural signs of human growth by The Nei Jung

According to the Nei Jung, commonly known as the Bible of Eastern Medicine, there are natural growth signs in humans that are observed through Eastern medicine. For example, at around 8 years old for males and 7 years old for females, baby teeth are replaced by permanent teeth and hair becomes thicker.

According to the Nei Jung, commonly known as the Bible of Eastern Medicine, there are natural growth signs in humans that are observed through Eastern medicine practices. For example, at around 8 years old for males and 7 years old for females, baby teeth are replaced by permanent teeth and hair becomes thicker.

Many parents are concerned about the pandemic due to the lack of information available.

Harold clinic

First check the mouth breathing second check the digestion poop pee must

Always goes together the priority is digestion see the first chapter

Early childhood trauma can have lasting negative effects on health, leaving individuals more vulnerable to disease and premature death. A high score on the Adverse Childhood Experiences (ACE) scale indicates the severity of trauma experienced.

Healing from trauma can be a challenging journey, often requiring the help of a trained therapist for the best support.

For example

Three-year-old rhinitis goes to eighty. If children have a yellow runny nose and a stuffy nose, there is a possibility that it is acute sinus, not a cold, so you should get detailed medical attention."

Many kids in hospital visit breathing issue
Parents many trouble to fine the answer kid

I think it is important to activate the right path get antigen naturally not by pill but by changing body temp or fresh food, air it heal by itself by wisdom of body Cause your kid have a miracle system that mother nature endow so check the breathing sleep and fresh food must

"Male 16 years old, female 14 years old, reproductive organs develop and it becomes possible for the woman to become pregnant. Sperm becomes abundant."with the onset of puberty, pregnancy becomes possible, sperm quantity increases.

"Female 21 years old, male 24 years old, growth of the body reaches its peak, and physical growth is at its maximum. Permanent teeth are fully developed.", growth in height is stabilized and growth reaches its peak, true teeth are fully formed.

One example

Director Lee posted a story about a high school patient more than 20 years ago. The student is an aspiring student at the Air Force Academy, but the passing of the physical fitness test was unclear due to severe sinust. At that time, it was not uncommon to have sincus surgery on teenagers, but Director Lee was cured by undergoing the first sinus endoscopic surgery introduced at the time. After that, the student became a construction cadet, and later became a state-of-the-art fighter pilot. The nose is pierced, so life is pierced. Director Lee said, "The nose is a gatekeeper that protects respiratory health, so active treatment also improves lung diseases such as asthma and bronchitis."

Sinus endoscopic surgery is a surgical procedure used to treat sinus-related conditions. This procedure involves the use of an endoscope, which is a thin, flexible tube with a camera and light source attached to it. The endoscope is inserted into the nose to allow the surgeon to visualize the inside of the sinus cavity. With the help of small instruments, the surgeon is able to remove any blockages, such as polyps or inflamed tissue, and improve the drainage of mucus from the sinuses. This surgery is considered a minimally invasive procedure, as it is performed through the nostrils and does not require any external incisions. The recovery time for sinus endoscopic surgery is typically shorter compared to traditional sinus surgery, and the risk of complications is generally lower. Overall, sinus endoscopic surgery is an effective treatment option for individuals with chronic sinusitis or other sinus-related conditions.

One of the three patients with similar symptoms to a cold is a child under the age of nine," said. "Children with atopic or asthma are more likely to develop allergic rhinitis, and these diseases last a lifetime, so don't think it will get better later, and you should thoroughly manage rhinitis from a young age," Lee said.

When asked about "life therapy that helps to reduce uncomfortable nose symptoms such as nasal congestion, sneezing, cough, and runny nose," Director Lee said, "The best nose health method recommended by an ototlaryngologist is to wash the nose." He said, "I wash the nasal cavity in the nose with menstrual saline water, and if you habitually brush your nose once or twice a day, you will give less than half the time to meet an otolaryngologist."

Kids and children have to learn about nutrition, cooking, and nature. Cooking can be a great choice for a job, especially for those who enjoy working with heat, like a chef. It is important for them to understand their body's constitution and how to maintain it. Cooking by themselves can be an educational experience, as they can learn about different foods while shopping for groceries. It is important for them to eat garlic, ginger, apple, onion, lemon, and lime with every meal to promote gut health and fight off infections. Occasionally eating fast food is acceptable, as long as they understand the need to detox afterwards.

Parents note

The most critical time for infection growth is a very crucial moment where choices are made.

It is important to educate oneself on all aspects of sickness, including the reasons, when and how to react, and to write memos about it.

Why constantly repeat these patterns throughout one's life. Therefore, it is crucial to provide the right information until they become accustomed to it, keep it in the medical history

It is important to know the symptoms, when and where they occur.

Sometimes there is hard to find answer the disease the cosmic energy is not favor to your kid

Case study 2

Terry, who is six years old, and Ryan, who is four years old, were spending more time on antibiotics than off. "We are willing to try anything," they said. They also mentioned that they liked their pediatrician, but felt that he only knew how to prescribe drugs. Both boys were well developed and appeared to be healthy except for their susceptibility to upper respiratory and ear infections.

the excessive use of antibiotics can actually worsen the problem it is meant to alleviate.

This is because it weakens the immune system and allows for the development of more and stronger resistant germs.

they reserve antibiotics for very severe infections only, after trying other remedies.

how to use echinacea, which is an herbal immune enhancer and antibiotic substitute made from the root of a native American plant called Echinacea purpurea (purple coneflower). It is nontoxic and readily available in health food stores. As general preventive measures, I recommended excluding milk and milk products from the boys' diet, giving them daily doses of vitamin C, and taking them to an osteopath who specializes in cranial therapy to relieve any breathing restrictions

Antibiotics are powerful tools for containing susceptible infections but must be reserved for instances where they are really
needed. The frequent use of antibiotics is not wise. In case of recurrent or chronic infections, it is important to increase natural resistance. Disease-causing germs are always present, but by enhancing immunity and natural healing capacity it is possible to reduce the chance that they can harm us.

When your kids are sick, what choice will you make? Will you wait for their system to naturally regain its function, to educate your kids about the importance of eating whole foods and fruits that are necessary for their health

or will you choose a quick solution that may temporarily affect and cause damage?
Teach them this knowledge for their entire lives, not just temporarily.

"Female 28 years old, male 32 years old, muscles and skeletal structure become more solid, reaching a complete stage." muscles and skeletal system become stronger, completing the growth process.

It's important to know your genetic risk factors
Understand your risk factors and talk to your primary doc. And realize that you can change see the 5 elementary chapter 3
Toxins: Abandon all tobacco (cigarettes, pipes, cigars). Why is smoking is bad for breathing make it simple tabacco reduce body heat

meaning make blood vessel contracting so high blood pressure is a little okay for reduce the heat

But most lung issue case need blood vessel expanding for circulation

Again regarding the toxic reaction of human body
first reaction is very important rejecting by instinct
but you do it again your immune is get less react toxic build up in your lung
just one time stress out is okay but it goes on you have to pay later on with high interest
You harm your financial life if you borrow $100,000 to work in a (perhaps interesting and noble) field
where you will realistically earn $20,000 a year, as more than half of your gross income will need to go to repay your debt over 10 years.
The same cancer toxic builds up you do not realize
you have to pay over 10 years more pain more harder when you getting old so

You need Backup plans for your health

"Male 40 years old, female 35 years old, three yanmyung meridian weaken li st
St and li li call the toxic and breathing

vital energy and meridian lose strength, kidney function declines, and teeth and hair deteriorate." vital energy weakens, the function of the skeletal system weakens, and teeth and hair deteriorate.

"Male 48 years old, female 42 years old, vitality declines, and hair becomes gray or white."
, energy declines and hair turns grey.

"Female 49 years old, male 56 years old, reproductive energy weakens, and vitality declines. Liver function weakens and sperm production decreases." veins weaken, pulse weakens, liver function declines, and sperm quantity decreases."

Harold's Treatment Plan by Age Group:
Males: 8 to 24 years
Females: 7 to 21 years

To assess health, evaluate the basic five-organ constitution and follow a natural approach that emphasizes proper diet and exercise, avoiding medication.

Key Inquiry:

What is the weakest organ? This organ is likely responsible for recurring symptoms.

Males: 25 to 48 years
Females: 22 to 42 years

Treatment for this age group focuses on balancing mixed health conditions, where some organs may exhibit hyperactive symptoms while others show signs of deficiency. Diagnosis should be made using the eight-pattern differentiation method.

Individuals Over 56 Years (Men) and Over 49 Years (Women):

Patients in this age bracket are more susceptible to aggravation and adverse effects during treatment due to depleted Kidney Yang, primordial Qi, and blood. Recovery may take longer; therefore, treatment should start with fundamental approaches to invigorate the functions of the kidneys, spleen, and liver.

An in-depth conversation about your physical, mental, and spiritual medical history is essential to determine the seriousness of your condition.

Western view

Middle forties to early seventies

Experts are just beginning to realize that balance starts to deteriorate in midde age. The changes are so subtle, and arrive so gradually, that they'te hart to spot unless you're looking for them. Most women aren't aware of balance problems during these years.

Mid-seventies and older

As small changes mount up, loss of balance begins to affect the quality of life. Active women notice the difference in demanding leisure activities such as biking, skiing, or running. Sedentary women feel less steady when they walk; they slow down, aware that they may fall.

One of the saddest consequences of deteriorating balance, aside from falling itself, is the fear of falling. This starts a vicious cycle that diminishes the quality of life. An older person becomes cautious physically--and rightly so. But this can lead to inactivity, weakness, and falls; the falls, in turn, prompt more fear and even less activity. For example, the patient's mother is eighty-five years old and experienced a fall last week. She was standing when she suddenly fell from her full height onto the paved driveway. She scraped her arms and legs, but fortunately, there was no internal damage or broken bones. However, she has lost her confidence and is now hesitant to go outside. I anticipate that I will need to move in with her.

"Virus Vulnerability by Age Group" by Anthony Williams

You may begin to notice symptoms in your 50s or 60s. These variations may partially persist in the thyroid, releasing only a few of their viral cells to inflame the nerves, which leads to relatively mild nerve inflammation. The only variety of EBV that medical communities are aware of is in this group.

EBV Group 3 will transition between stages faster than Group 2, so its symptoms might be noticeable around age 40. Also, these viruses fully complete Stage Four--that is, they entirely leave the thyroid to latch onto nerves. Viruses in this group can cause a variety of ills, including joint pain, fatigue, heart palpitations, tinnitus, and vertigo.

EBV Group 4 will create noticeable problems as early as age 30.
Its aggressive actions on nerves can result in symptoms associated with fibromyalgia, chronic fatigue syndrome, brain fog, confusion, anxiety, moodiness, and everything caused by Groups 1 to 3. This group can also create symptoms of posttraumatic stress disorder, even if a person never underwent any trauma beyond getting inflamed by the virus.

EBV Group 5 will create noticeable issues as early as age 20. This is an especially nasty form of the virus because it strikes just when a young person is setting out to start an independent life. It can create all the problems of Group 4, and it feeds off negative emotions such as fear and worry. Doctors who can't find anything wrong, and perceive these patients as young and healthy, often declare "it's all in your head" and send them to psychologists to convince them what's actually happening in their bodies isn't real. Unless, that is, a patient happens upon a doctor who's up on the Lyme disease trend, in which case the patient will probably walk away with a Lyme misdiagnosis.

The worst type, however, is EBV Group 6, which can strike hard even in young children. In addition to everything Group 5 does, Group 6 can create symptoms so severe that they're misdiagnosed as leukemia, viral meningitis, lupus, and more. Plus it suppresses the immune system, which can lead to a wide variety of

There is evidence that capillaries, as well as arteries, may experience impaired functions as individuals age.

Capillaries and interstitial colloid.

I appreciate the crucial yet often unseen role of capillaries in our bodies, especially in relation to the lymphatic system, which also operates invisibly to help combat viruses.

There is evidence that capillaries, as well as arteries, may experience impaired functions as individuals age. In a histological examination of muscles conducted by Buccianti and Luria, it was discovered that interstitial colloid accumulates in older individuals and the elastic tissue surrounding the muscle fibers becomes thicker. Capillaries are located in this region between the muscle fibers. When additional material is present between the capillaries and the muscle cells, it becomes evident that the capillaries would not be able to efficiently carry out their function, even if they dilate when the muscle becomes active. This is because the diffusion of respiratory gases, particularly oxygen, which has a relatively slow diffusion rate, would encounter obstacles.

Interstitial colloid refers to a substance or material that is present in the interstitial space of a tissue or organ. This substance helps to maintain the integrity and function of the cells and tissues by providing support and cushioning. The interstitial colloid is composed of proteins and other molecules that help to regulate the flow of fluids and nutrients within the tissue. It also plays a key role in the immune response and the removal of waste products from the cells. Overall, the interstitial colloid is an essential component of the extracellular matrix and is vital for the overall health and function of the body.

Capillaries are tiny blood vessels that are responsible for connecting arteries and veins. They play a crucial role in the circulation of blood throughout the body. Capillaries have thin, permeable walls that allow for the exchange of nutrients, oxygen, and waste products from the bloodstream to the surrounding tissues. They are also involved in the regulation of blood flow and pressure. Capillaries can be found in all parts of the body, including the lungs, digestive system, and muscles.

Cognitive function changes due to aging

Changes in cognitive function due to aging vary from person to person, and the speed at which cognitive function declines also varies by cognitive domain. A large-scale study tracking changes in cognitive function due to aging in the United States was conducted. Known as the 'Seattle Longitudinal Study', it was initiated by Washington University in Seattle in 1956. Over 50 years, the study surveyed more than 6,000 individuals aged 20 to 90, analyzing language fluency, reasoning abilities, memory, spatial and visual perception, numerical abilities, and speed of recognizing specific signals.

The results showed that cognitive function peaks in the 30s to 40s and gradually declines with age. However, speed of cognitive perception peaks at age 25 and continues to decline thereafter. Numerical abilities decline significantly starting from the 60s, placing them at the lowest level among the 6 cognitive abilities surveyed. Age is just a number, but it is true that cognitive abilities weaken as we age.

Inference ability, language ability, and spatial perception ability are better for people in their 50s compared to those in their 20s and 30s. However, they decline in their late 60s. Language ability tends to remain relatively stable until around the age of 80, but then declines rapidly in the mid-80s. Even in their late 80s, language ability tends to be preserved compared to other cognitive abilities.

There are two types of intelligence: fluid and crystal. Fluid intelligence refers to the ability to solve problems and learn new ways of abstracting. Crystal intelligence refers to the ability to use acquired and accumulated knowledge. According to a longitudinal study in Seattle, fluid intelligence tends to decrease with age while crystal intelligence tends to improve. This means that while adaptability may decline with age, judgment and reasoning remain intact.

There is a theory of brain plasticity, suggesting that the brain changes shape as it is used, just like clay. The more the brain is used, the more its functions are activated. Nowadays, the physical capacity of elderly individuals has improved significantly compared to the time of the Seattle longitudinal study, so it is expected that cognitive function related to aging has also declined less. Our brains continue to develop, and the rate of aging has slowed down

Longevity is a leading topic in the current health community.

I would like to share three inspiring longevity cases with you. One is from the United States, while the other two are from Japan, where many people live to be over 100 years old.

Case 1)

Internal medicine doctor Hinoharashi Segiaki, who led the "Shinno Inu (New Elderly)" movement in Japan, lived a respectable life until he passed away at the age of 106. When

He gave more than 100 lectures a year and his health practices are still being followed four years after his passing. Last year, the famous US economic broadcasting station CNBC covered the "Hinoharashi-style secrets to living in the 100-year-old era".

He emphasized 10 rules for a healthy long life. The key message was not just living long, but living meaningfully. He stressed the importance of living life to the fullest until the moment of death. Even in retirement, he advocated for engaging in social service. Until a few months before his passing, he worked up to 18 hours a day.

He said that those who love and are loved live longer and emphasized the importance of always creating and living for others. This passage makes one think about why longevity is important. He also believed that difficulties in life are the same everywhere, so one should create a welcoming home and have active social interactions. He advised paying attention to the interests of young people and making laugh lines on our faces. A positive attitude and harmony are the keys to longevity.

He said that loving and being loved a lot leads to a long and healthy life. He also emphasized constantly creating and living for the sake of others. This is the part that makes one think about why they should live a long life. He then said that difficult things in life are the same everywhere, so one should create a home where people easily come and interact with others. He also mentioned paying attention to the interests of young people and laughing to create wrinkles on one's face.

He said that a positive attitude and harmony are the secrets to longevity.

He also recommended constantly using one's body. He always took the stairs and stepped on two steps at once. He said that the biggest obstacle to elderly health is falling and breaking bones, so he advised practicing falling safely, where muscles in the buttocks would touch the ground before the rest of the body, before going to bed.

Lastly, he advised having a doctor who listens to the patient. He said that doctors should not be seen as all-knowing, and that culture and art are necessary for joy and inner peace. He mentioned that enjoying something is the best way to forget pain.

Case 2)

The average body mass index (BMI) of Sato is 23.9, with a body fat percentage of 25% and muscle mass of 44.6 kg. She is a healthy woman in her 30s. The health center suspected machine malfunction and checked her several times. How is this possible? Last month, I met Sato Hide from Iwate Prefecture, which is 500 km away from Tokyo in the northeast direction.

Sato laughed when I came to ask about the secret of "99 years old and still going strong".she wakes up at 6 am every morning, listens to the radio while doing exercises, and during the day, he moves his hands on a sewing machine to make dolls or reform clothes. When she is not moving her body, he reads magazines with small letters called "Naan".

I saw the bleakness of "living" and at the same time, I felt the nobility of "living.""

"A typical day's routine:

"I wake up at 6 am every day. After making my bed and preparing breakfast in advance, at 6:30 I do the 'Radio Exercise' to the NHK radio broadcast. I take my time eating breakfast and always watch the NHK morning drama. At 9:30, I start making dolls. I clean the house every day. I also vacuum every 2-3 days. I personally cook and eat three meals every day, and I eat quite a lot (laughs). Whenever I go grocery shopping twice a week, I buy a lot of vegetables. For breakfast, I eat rice and soup with fish and meat, and I also eat natto (fermented soybean food). I go to bed around 11 pm. Before going to bed, around 10 pm, I take a bath and do about 500 kicks in the water."

"Do you eat protein every day?"

"I eat fish and meat regularly. I buy dried fish and freeze it. Usually, I grill it to eat. I don't really like deep-fried fish because of the oil."

Separate exercise. "I don't do any special exercise, but since this is the second floor, I go up and down the stairs. The internal medicine doctor says that if you want to live until 100 years old, you should climb about 6 floors of stairs, but it's impossible for me because my house is only 2 floors. I take walks back and forth near my house. I want to take walks on the main road, but there are no benches to sit and rest in the middle, so I can't go. I feel a little bit of my old age in situations like this."

- Do you go to the hospital regularly?

"I go to Day Service (daytime care service) every Friday. I bring my nephew and daughter-in-law who has dementia when I turned 70. At the Day Service, they check body temperature, do light exercises, and do brain exercises like paper folding, and they learn a lot. It's free time during the day, but other elderly people take naps or chat, but I find it a waste of time so I learn to reform clothes during this time. I started this new job around the age of 88."

I fall asleep quickly.

"I take deep breaths five times while lying in bed. A posture correction teacher told me that it is good to expand my chest, so I am making an effort to do so. I fall asleep right after deep breath. Sometimes I wake up at night, but I usually go back to sleep after going to the bathroom. I sleep for about 7 hours a day. Before bed, I don't use my cellphone and I sleep with the curtains closed to make it dark.

- They say it's also good to read newspapers and magazines.

"I subscribe to a monthly magazine called 'Jichi'. When it is delivered, I read it all at once, and sometimes I read it again when I have free time. I also read when I don't feel like sewing or when I am a little tired. The reason I read magazines is to supplement my knowledge and have enjoyable conversations with friends. I often meet up with people around me and also make phone calls. I have more than 10 conversation partners."

"Do you drink alcohol and smoke?

"I enjoy occasionally drinking beer with young people. Seeing young people enjoy beer, I tried it too. Nowadays, I drink one can of beer while watching dramas 2-3 times a week in the evening."

-Is your weight stable? Do you take any health supplements?

"I have maintained a weight of 60-65kg throughout my life. I don't take any health supplements. Wouldn't it be better to have a proper meal rather than relying on supplements?

Recently, I even tried instant ramen for the first time in my life. I gave some clothes I tailored to an acquaintance, and they gave me instant ramen as a thank-you gift. It tasted good. However, it had a lot of salt, so I didn't drink the soup. I also don't drink the soup when eating udon or soba. But I drink the soup when I make soybean paste soup. It is made with good soybean paste from a well-known store, so it's fine.

I prefer tea over coffee and eat fruit every day. I also drink wine and eat ice cream. Doctors say I shouldn't, but I still eat desserts because they taste delicious (laughs)."

Case 3)

.Marissa Teijo, a 70-year-old woman who drew attention by participating in the Miss Universe USA beauty pageant in the United States, revealed the secret to maintaining her youth in an interview with the US media People on the 23rd (local time).

Marissa Teijo, who was the "oldest contestant ever" in Miss Universe USA, said about her diet, "I mainly eat vegetables, fruits, and oatmeal," and added, "I occasionally enjoy chicken, fish, steak, and other meat."

Teijo said, "I don't eat cheese, processed meat (ham, sausage, etc.), or white bread," and explained, "I enjoy indulging in cookies made with almond flour and a little sugar."

Teijo also mentioned that she exercises regularly, stating, "I started strength training at the age of 40 and did it about 5-6 days a week. I used to do running and aerobics consistently, but when I started strength training, my body began to change. Developing muscles in the upper body made my waist look slimmer."

She recently reduced her strength training as she aged but said that she still engages in aerobic exercises like walking on the remaining days. Teijo emphasized the importance of staying active, saying, "I am very active. I don't stop. This is one of the strong recommendations I give to everyone," and added, "Just don't stop. If you keep moving, you will be able to move well even as you age."

In response to the question about what beauty means to her, Teijo said, "Sharing happiness and joy, treating others kindly gives me energy and beauty," and continued, "This becomes an attractive quality that draws people in."

She also expressed her belief that having confidence regardless of appearance or physique is another form of beauty.

The Texas USA pageant took place last month. Although Teijo did not win an award, her participation brought hope to middle-aged and older women.

Acupuncture

Eastern medicine emphasizes three main principles in the clinic: First comes acupuncture, followed by moxibustion, and finally herbal treatment.

When using acupuncture, it is recommended to use the smallest needle possible. In my clinic, I commonly use a general size of 0.18 by 30 mm, but a smaller size of 0.16 by 15 mm can be used for specific areas such as the face, to address issues like toothaches, wrinkles, hearing problems, and eye conditions. Inserting the needle before sleeping can effectively help alleviate these symptoms.

There is no need to be afraid when using acupuncture. Simply place the needle on your own pain points or areas of discomfort, such as your neck, face, or shoulders. Specifically, try placing the needle on the tip of your nose and indang points for breathhing issue. You may notice positive effects in the morning.

Why is acupuncture the first option? After the pandemic, many Westerners are turning to learning Eastern medicine, including acupuncture, to address their own symptoms. It helps to make connections within the body, as all parts are interconnected. When symptoms suggest a breakdown in communication between different body parts, acupuncture can help by ensuring the flow of energy is restored.

Why is it that acupuncture can influence every myelin sheath of nerves, tapping into unseen energy pockets to accelerate nerve signals and facilitate capillary and lymphatic movement, thereby promoting overall wellness—even when these mechanisms are not visible? You may not always see the effects, but you can definitely feel them.

In Western medicine, the electrolytes in the brain are understood through complex chemical analyses, yet the concept can be simplified by likening it to a wire being disconnected by a virus. Why is the function of myelinated nerves so important? Most nerve damage occurs in these areas, and while Western medicine often resorts to surgeries with advanced equipment, the reality is that such interventions may leave permanent damage behind. The invisible energy pockets created by nature are not meant to be analyzed; rather, they require the same invisible energy input, whether it's through heat, magnets, or acupuncture, to facilitate healing and recovery from a virus. Instead of directly targeting the virus, the focus should be on restoring the energy of the myelin sheath.

Another benefit of acupuncture is that it has no side effects. and can be done by anyone, anywhere, at any time. When you're tired or struggling with insomnia, you need a mind-body connection. The best time for acupuncture is during REM sleep, when lymph flow is abundant and the body's natural healing powers are at their peak. Inserting tiny needles at specific points on the body and tapping them lightly can provide pain relief and promote healing by connecting to the body's internal systems through meridian channels.

Acupuncture may not kill viruses, but it helps circulate lymph fluids to fight back naturally.

Some recently western doctor work together eastern doctor before surgery or after surgery

Combined treatment

an acupuncture point is referred to as the "junction of the human rivers."

these points are meeting points or intersections on the meridians, symbolizing the flow of energy through the body resembling rivers.

Our bodies simply know what to do; we don't need to analyze the wisdom of the body. Just relax

You'll know it's working when you feel it; you don't have to prove anything by feeling good. The best doctor is yourself, as only you know your symptoms and feelings. You can do this by yourself, so trust your instincts and choose the right needle.

Celebrity Jennifer Lawrence said

A good needling

"I have found acupuncture to be really, really helpful for soothing muscle stiffness, aches and pain,says Jennifer. "But I also use it more systemically to help balance my hormones, energy levels and even digestive system. If you look at your body like an ocean, there are tides coming in and out, and it could get really tumultuous. I've learned that acupuncture helps calm those waters." Jennifer adds, "Come to think of it,

When inserting a needle, one can feel a stiff and tense sensation at the tip of the needle, as if there is a thread attached. The patient feels a tingling sensation, similar to being electrically shocked, with a soothing and refreshing feeling.

In acupuncture, precise stimulation corresponding to the disease is obtained. The sensation of acupuncture treatment is more pleasurable rather than painful.

The sensation is achieved through the stimulation of nerves and blood vessels, but the distribution of visible nerves and blood vessels differs from the distribution pathway of sensation obtained through stimulation. This distribution pathway of sensation can be called as meridians.

Trigger Point Therapy for myofascial Pain

In reality, what is happening is that the injured nerves trigger the release of an "alarm" hormone to notify the body that the nerves are exposed and in need of repair.

A nerve is similar to a string of yarn with small root hairs hanging from it. When the nerve is injured, the root hairs detach from the sides of the nerve sheath. EBV searches for these openings and attaches itself to them.

In simpler terms, the nerve sheath is like a protective layer around the nerve, while nerve myelination refers to the coating that helps nerve signals travel faster.

The same doing the job acupuncture how

Neurons are cells that are capable of generating and conducting electrical impulses. These impulses are caused by the movement of sodium and potassium ions across the cell membrane.

Impulse it means the insert the needle The inside of neurons has a slightly negative charge compared to the outside, with a resting membrane potential between -50 and -80 millivolts (mV). This means the cell is electrically polarized.

This is a great tip to prevent all viruses from bursting out. There are lots of tiny nerves and vessels in the nose that require a tiny needle to address them. It's important to understand why a needle is needed. The root hair located in the nose only activates the mucus, causing lots of tears to burst out. This can still result in a sharp pain in the tip of the nose. However, after coughing four times, all the viruses are expelled and the lymph mucus begins to work effectively, which is a great progress. The area in the middle and top of the nose is the main concern.

To strengthen the defense mechanism, it is important to activate the mucus glands and lymph flow. This is where the effectiveness of using a needle lies. Simply insert the needle into the nose while sleeping, and you will see great results. The reason for using a tiny needle is to reactivate the lymph and mucus, and to detoxify the body.

First, the toxic blood is expelled by reactivating the lymph, along with white fluid. If you experience an itching sensation in your throat, you can also use the needle in the throat to achieve clear voice and clear breathing. This is a great idea for improving the oxygen intake.

Acupuncture close to the bone, rather than in the middle of the muscle, targets the motor and sensory nerves that originate from the connective tissue in the bone. This means that acupuncture near the bone or directly on the bone itself can alleviate pain and other symptoms.

The connective tissue is the main trouble area and the core acupuncture points.that is the myophagia the same meaning it occur that hwa ta points the same
For the same reason, acupuncture needles must be placed close to the spinal cord.

Face acupuncture is also important because all cranial nerves pass through the face. Additionally, the Eastern stomach meridian, as well as SI, LI, GB, triple burner, pericardium, and conceptional and du meridians, pass through the face.

Also woman wrinkle and cosmetic treatment is great for acupuncture in that case more small need is effective best time is rem sleep so before go to bed put the needle in wrinkle point insert the needle that is all

You will see in the morning

In practice, when dealing with the Western 11 cranial nerve, simply touching different areas of the face to find the pain point is sufficient. Once the main point is identified, the needle should be inserted slowly and gently. If a sharp pain occurs, the needle should be stopped, and after 15 minutes, the pain should be checked again. If it has disappeared, the needle can be inserted further to a deeper level.

The best time to insert the needle is before sleep, allowing the body to naturally heal itself. When you wake up, check the area for any bleeding, which indicates the release of toxins.

To embark on our healing journey, it is essential to seek the right guidance from professionals who understand both the physical and mental aspects of our well-being. Our bodies are not linear systems; they are dynamic and continuously evolving at a cellular level.

So, how can we adapt to these changes? The key is to listen to ourselves, as we carry over 80% of the responsibility for identifying the root causes of our issues and selecting appropriate healing methods. Healing is not a one-time event; it requires ongoing commitment, even during sleep, in addition to meditation, nutrition, and adequate oxygen.

We must thoughtfully evaluate the numerous treatment options available to us, as simple chronic conditions or viruses cannot be effectively addressed with a single remedy; they require a comprehensive, multi-faceted approach.

Simple put it

You can obtain a wealth of information from the 365 acupuncture points, which represent a comprehensive approach to addressing a variety of symptoms. To understand the underlying issues, it is essential to examine the five major organs and the six fu organs.

Acupuncture can be utilized on various parts of the body, including the lungs (for breathing), the skull, the nose, the face, the neck and shoulders, as well as the gut.

Many diseases originate in the gut, which is why numerous viruses, including proviruses, thrive there. The gut is subjected to daily exposure, making it highly susceptible to infections, and it is one of the most complex systems that goes beyond laboratory testing.

When inserting a needle, you can feel a tense tension as if there is a thread at the tip of the needle, with a smooth and short insertion. Patients feel a sharp and exhilarating sensation, as if being electrocuted. The patient feels a tingling sensation, like being electrified, which is both refreshing and exciting.

Locally, an accurate sense of gain corresponding to the disease is obtained.

The feeling of gain from acupuncture can sometimes be felt as pleasure, and there is no pain during the acupuncture process.

The sense of gain is obtained by stimulating the nerves and blood vessels, but the distribution of visible nerves and blood vessels and the distribution line of sensory perception obtained by stimulation are different. This pathway of sensory perception can be called the meridian.

Blood flow is crucial for activating brain functions and mental activities. It is also essential for overall health. The fewer needles used during treatments, the better, and around 10 needles are usually appropriate.

Yintang (GV29)

Japanese tiny moxibustion

Japanese tiny moxibustion are effective options for treating virus diseases. Moxibustion involves the use of mugwort that has been aged for at least 3 years, typically 5 years. This aging process transforms it into a potent medicinal material that interacts well with the body's temperature, making it suitable and effective.

Although moxibustion may cause temporary scarring on the skin, it typically heals within 1-2 weeks.

Why is moxibustion effective against viruses? It is simple because viruses can only be killed by heat.

Recent evidence has shown the vulnerability of bedbugs to heat.

Bedbugs can survive for up to one day without feeding on blood. Despite being able to withstand temperatures as low as negative 20 degrees for 30 minutes, they cannot survive temperatures exceeding 50 degrees due to their sensitivity to heat. Bedbugs can be effectively controlled by exposing them to high temperatures.

Bedbugs have a sensitivity to heat and cannot survive in temperatures exceeding 50 degrees. They can withstand cold temperatures for a short period but are effectively controlled by exposure to high heat.

Bedbugs thrive between the months of September and December when the temperature ranges from 18 to 20 degrees. Professor Yang Young-cheol from Eulji University stated, "The ideal temperature for their rapid growth is around 27 to 28 degrees," and "It takes only 36 days for them to hatch from an egg and reach adulthood." Unlike mosquitoes, bedbugs do not possess efficient blood-sucking abilities, resulting in bites occurring in two to three successive spots, often forming a circular pattern. They commonly reside in beds, mattresses, and similar areas where humans sleep and provide a blood source.

The same principle to the virus including covid virus
They never die just kill or be killed of breathing patients
This moxa heat up to 60 degrees sustain 3 minutes increased the dramatically the red blood cell circulation

At the age of 89, she operates an acupuncture clinic in Japan alongside her son, who is also an acupuncturist. She mentioned that there are no side effects associated with this natural healing method. Although she focuses exclusively on acupuncture, her son specializes in moxibustion, which complements their practice and benefits their elderly patients. An elderly individual in Japan practiced this daily at ST 36 to improve his digestion problem, which proved to be effective.

Most of back pain loss of connection loss of metabolism loss of narrow the nerve and blood vessel all that from the shrinking lower function of it
So apply heat simple to expanding or activate
It Is the main concept of the functional medicine

Moxibustion is the most effective way to enhance body function, eliminate viruses that may be dormant inside of you, and address issues such as inflammation, scar tissue, or nerve pain, particularly in the neuro or nervous system.

How to do that

Simple put it

Virus covered Toxic protein layer called **Encapsulating itself**

High heat the melting the calcification of virus layer feeding pure your blood

Most case is stage 3 4 cancer

heat increase metabolism to cover debt oxygen debt energy

finally thick toxic blood coming out it is the final treat killing virus

Virus doing **Encapsulating itself** into the inactive cyst form

referring to the concept of a cyst in a dormant or inactive state. In biology, a cyst is a protective structure formed by certain organisms, such as bacteria, fungi, protozoa, or parasites, as a response to unfavorable conditions in their environment.

When a cyst is in an active or dormant state, i the organism within the cyst is actively growing, replicating, or carrying out metabolic processes.

Through the western medical history

cannot be cured by a knife can be cured by fire, by cauterization (burning or searing of the wounds)

also good for A blood clot,

also known as a thrombus, is a gel-like mass formed by the clumping of platelets and clotting factors in the blood. Blood clots can occur in the veins (deep vein thrombosis) or arteries, leading to potential complications. Symptoms of a blood clot may include swelling, pain, redness, and warmth in the affected area. Blood clots can be serious, especially if they break loose and travel through the bloodstream to vital organs.

It is basic point that legendary south Korea master point out two points to treat digestion and cold symptom most is the basic symptom of clinic most patinets have

ST 36 for digestion lower point of stomach and LU 7 is the treat the cold at the lung meridian

It cause a little scar happen I use the Vichy cream

Magnets therapy

First I am interesting magnets therapy personally after reading this article

A machine that prevents water stains in pipes is a magnetic device that creates a symmetrical magnetic field on both sides of the pipe. It removes water stains in long drainage pipes and extends the lifespan of boilers. Similarly, when a perpendicular magnetic field is applied to the flow of blood, which has better magnetic permeability than water, the blood becomes magnetized. Impurities in the blood are ionized and minerals are activated, and water molecules in the blood are activated, resulting in clean blood. Deposits such as cholesterol in blood vessels are also removed. However, this method of washing blood with magnets requires strong stimulation with magnets applied to the fingers or ankles. The use of magnets for necklaces or other skin contact is not based on the principle of blood washing, but solely on the stimulation effect. For this specific method of washing blood with magnets, special magnets with at least 2,000 gauss or more are required. Blood becomes electrified when the magnetic field lines penetrate through the blood vessels to the opposite side.

I did research all western eastern point of view

The earliest known use of magnetism is the compass. Compasses use magnetized
needles to indicate which direction is north. They have been used in navigation for hundreds of years.

how to migrate the bird?
seasonal bird flow magnet field

Have you ever observed a cat or a dog in a state of relaxation?
They seem almost magnetically attached to the earth, with relaxed, soft, and tender bodies that breathe calmly without any signs of shortness of breath. There is minimal tension in their bodies, resulting in reduced oxygen needs.

Why?
The plasmasphere of Earth is an inner component of the magnetosphere and is situated outside the upper ionosphere in the Earth's atmosphere. It comprises a dense and cold plasma that envelops our planet. While plasma exists throughout the magnetosphere, the plasmasphere typically contains the coldest plasma.

Plasma emits light through a process called "spontaneous emission," which occurs when ions, atoms, or molecules possess a higher energy level than stable ones, causing them to become unstable and emit photons.

See the quantum biology and magnet

How can quantum mechanical concepts be applicable to this physiological domain?
Quantum physicists are not concerned with shapes, but rather with fields. In quantum mechanics, molecules are not rigid stick-and-ball

entities with fixed angles, but rather entities where the electrons generate a force in one area, similar to a magnet.

In the 1770s, Franz Friedrich Anton Mesmer was a young doctor practicing medicine in Vienna when his life was forever changed by a chance encounter with a Jesuit priest named Maximilian Hell. Maximilian Hell, also known as Father Hell, was conducting medical experiments using magnetized lodestone plates. He applied these plates to the bodies of sick patients, hoping to provide relief for diseases like rheumatism. Mesmer was captivated by the priest's demonstrations and adopted Hell's magnetic theory, but he took it a step further, creating his own uniquely bizarre philosophy.

Mesmer believed that every single disease was caused by an imbalance in the body's universal magnetic fluid, which was susceptible to gravitational force. Initially, he thought that magnets could correct these imbalances. However, Mesmer soon became convinced that he possessed the true power to realign the magnetic fluids within himself.

He referred to this universal magnetic fluid as "animal magnetism." Mesmer believed that by laying his hands on patients and exerting his willpower, he could manipulate this fluid and heal the sick.

The concept that human bodies contained a mysterious, universal fluid that could be influenced by external forces was not new. In fact, it was like the way light filters in through stained glass windows in the spacious saloon.

All the walls in the room are adorned with mirrors, enhancing its aesthetic appeal. The pleasant scent of orange blossoms wafts through the air, creating a soothing atmosphere. In the distance, the gentle singing and the melodious strumming of a harp can be heard.

I used the NorthSouth Biomagnetics magnetic mattress and magnetic bars. After a small moxa treatment, I placed small pieces of magnets on the scar which resulted in a lot of lymph fluids being released, indicating a significant detoxification process. I also applied magnets to the nose and placed them behind the ear, targeting the limbic system to enhance the production of sleep molecules.

Magnetic therapy helps in balancing free radicals and improving lymphatic flow. It is observed that body fluids and free radicals tend to be more acidic in type 2 individuals, while those with a higher metal and water content tend to experience better REM sleep when magnets are utilized effectively.

Through the clinic, I believe there is great potential for the lymphatic system to cleanse the body of waste and reactivating the lymph. Additionally, placing it at the tip of the nose can heal the nasal mucous membrane, which is very impressive. I highly recommend using it in conjunction with acupuncture and magnetic therapy in the nose.

The magnetic field generated by the magnets harmonizes free radical fluids in the body. Atoms consist of positively charged protons and neutral particles called neutrons in the nucleus, while negatively charged electrons orbit around them. Electrons have the ability to break away from the atom as they are not contained within the nucleus.

A magnetic field creates an invisible area around the magnet, influencing the pH balance within the body.

Again
the blood's pH level influences the respiratory rate. When the blood becomes more acidic, the respiration rate increases to eliminate excess CO_2 and restore pH balance. Conversely, when the blood becomes more

alkaline, the respiration rate decreases to allow for a buildup of CO2, aiding in lowering the pH.

There are two general sources of acid/base imbalances termed respiratory acidosis/alkalosis or metabolic/renal acidosis/alkalosis based on the cause of the imbalance.

Earthing is often helpful to reduce the electrical charge load. The idea here is for the body to come in direct contact with the ground via a conducting
medium - for example, walking barefoot on grass, earth, rock, etc. Wearing rubber-soled shoes or boots blocks this effect.

Secret to Making Self Appear with Fingers

Why finger again all connecting heavenly energy as we see the meridian theory

The right thum finger emits magnetic fields of the north pole, while the 3rd finger middle fnger the left index finger emits magnetic fields of the south pole.
Fingers of young practitioners emit a lot of magnetism.
When these fingers are placed near the north and south poles of a magnet, there is a healing effect like igniting a fire.
People with exceptional magnetic abilities can perform miraculous treatments where paralysis is instantly cured as soon as the fingers are applied."

Magnetic needle

Clinic case

"We expose the worst case of relieving headaches for our husband. We hope it will be helpful to someone suffering from headaches. The acupoints used for stimulation are 2 points (deep space between the bone connecting the fourth toe and the bone connecting the little toe).

First, steam the sides of the body, corresponding to the gallbladder meridian, until the headache improves. Keeping the body warm is to circulate the energy. Also, sticker needles are needed. If you search for 'magnetic needles' on the internet, you can find sticker needles with 1mm needles attached to round magnets for home use. Apply two sticker needles on each foot, a total of four.

First, apply the sticker needle. Every 30 minutes for two hours, lightly tap with the thumb and index finger to stimulate. Remove and disinfect after 2 hours. Then, apply the sticker needle without much stimulation and remove and disinfect after 8 hours.

When my husband applies magnetic needles, the pain suddenly disappears after 2 hours. It's not always the case, as on some days, after removing the sticker he falls asleep comfortably after 2 hours. When he complains of stiff side, applying sticker needles and lying down for a while make his body comfortable. As these incidents happen frequently, my husband is not interested in other acupoints, just remembers2 points and always presses and sleeps when his body is not feeling well."

Bloodletting and lancet pin

Another topic related to blood detox is the popular use of the Lancet pin

These were the theories of Hippocrates and his belief in the four humors. Whether it was an excess of blood, phlegm, yellow bile, or black bile, the solution was often to purge the body through bleeding, vomiting, or clearing the bowels.

Even Erasistratus, who didn't support bloodletting, unintentionally popularized the practice in the third century BC by suggesting that many illnesses were caused by an overload of blood. Despite his recommendations of vomit-inducing, dietary changes, or exercise to treat blood overload, many doctors resorted to bloodletting. It was only a matter of time before this practice became a cure-all.

In the second century CE, Galen declared that bleeding was the answer to any bodily ailment, including hemorrhages. It is astonishing to think about how limited our understanding of anatomy and physiology was at that time. Bloodletting was often performed in a reasonable manner, avoiding young children and the elderly or refraining from excessive removal.

The main treat is like stage 4 or 3 In case of disease needle top of moxa is apply and toxic blood out by burning the tissue

a turning point occurred with the use of the Lancet pin. It was discovered that by pricking a small amount of blood, it effectively treated spasms and improved blood circulation in the bones and ligaments,

Firstly, bloodletting is not just a way to supply oxygen, it also helps to unclog the blood vessels. The lancet pin is essential for this procedure. In emergency situations like high blood pressure or stroke, bloodletting is needed immediately, ideally within 4 minutes. Furthermore, bloodletting is also beneficial for children during their growth period as it helps reduce excess heat. Overall, bloodletting is crucial because it ensures clean blood circulation and aids in oxygen delivery, as well as performing the function of killing viruses and disconnecting them from the food. The question remains, how can we effectively accomplish this procedure?

Why is it important? Virus needs food. It feeds on toxic blood, not in the bloodstream. It sucks up pure blood from the blood veins, which is your nutrition. However, regular blood tests won't be able to detect it. Your blood is being stolen and you don't even realize it. The nutrition you consume is not all for you; some of it is feeding the virus. The virus thrives in different stages, forming colonies in layers. Bloodletting is the process that reverses this, removing the toxic blood that feeds the virus. Western blood is the infection itself, but this is not widely recognized.

A certain doctor in Japan discovered a secret remedy for cardiac arrest called Soko. It is said that by removing a few drops of blood from the fingers or nails of a newborn experiencing cardiac arrest using a needle at the base on both sides of the fifth finger's fingernail, many lives can be saved.

removing a few drops of blood from under the fifth finger's fingernail with a needle can save many lives.

Here is the thing small drop of toxic blood with lancet pin needle

It is effective on the emergency and some excess hyper symptom or breathing stagnation

Also it is effective for kids and hyper blood pressure or emergency of stroke before call 911 more bloodletting in the back of neck imbue the oxygen to the brain already blood clogging accumulated so quick and fast you feel dangerous

So heart attack ams stroke must have a lancet pin needle for sure before emergency get an history of that disease call 911.

Chapter 3

5 elementary theories

5 elementary theories in the UK

The first person who played a significant role in introducing Eastern Medicine to the UK 120 years ago was the late J.L. Wolsley, a legendary acupuncturist in the UK. He was amazed to witness the use of anesthesia through the needle and immersed himself in the principles of Eastern Medicine

Nora Franglen, who is the Founder / Principal of the School of Five Element Acupuncture (SOFEA) in London says in her book "A study of the 5 elements" as abstract concepts is a study of the very essence of life itself. How then to find a way on to this vast landscape?

She learns under late J.R Wolsley, a legendary Acupuncturist Patterns of Practice Mastering the Art of Five Element Acupuncture The Simple Guide to Five Element Acupuncture as abstract concepts is a study of the very essence of life itself.

The Five Guardian Elements of Acupuncture: Custodians of the Soul

Endowing it with characteristics specific to the element all the elements flow to a rhythm within us, their interplay determining who we are

The combination of elements that goes to make up our individual that cannot be replicated elsewhere Element is of the causative factor of disease or the constitutional element. The CF causable factor thus becomes the primary focus for acupuncture treatment

This two-person vision is the reason why the clinic boutique available in the U.K. is so popular.

It offers western herbs and acupuncture, thus providing an advanced level of clinical service that combines Eastern and Western medicine techniques in the U.K.

This is not surprising given the increasing demand for such integrated medical approaches. Here nature comes to our aid, offering us evidence of the elements' one way in is to look at how the elements unfold through the cycles of our life we know of as our ageing process how the elements spread their spheres of influence over us through the medium of the organs of the body

Eastern medicine in the US

There are two American doctors who have shown an interest in Eastern Medicine in 1970. Peter Ackman obtained his medical degree, and his father was a surgeon. Erik, on the other hand, has a different perspective on the body system, influenced by the laws of the University and the five-organ diagnosis.

Peter Eckman (2007) author of "In the Footsteps of the Yellow Emperor", CF is that it is The Element of Official whose chronic state of imbalance cannot be completely corrected by nature itself, and which in turn is responsible for producing or at least allowing imbalances to develop and persist in the other Elements.

Another book by Ted Kaptchuk, author of *The Web That Has No Weaver*: *Between Heaven and Earth* by Harriet Beinfield, and Efrem Korngold

Author said, highlight the distinction between an intellectual, analytical approach (Talmudic intellect) and a more emotional, experiential approach (Hasidic soul) to practicing Judaism.

A WEB of interrelated things and events just as the sun maps out from distinct seasons in its yearly monthly so all biological organization go through four seasons in its yearly round Defined only by its function as part of the whole pattern

Western mind always the creator or cause and the phenomenon is merely its refection what is beyond behind or cause of there is an inherent truth or essence that exists within or is readily accessible within the nature of things.

Qi is the cause and also the effect basic stuff

Saying Five-Phase Theory: Evolutionary Stages of Transformation A Holographic Map Phases As Transformative Stages

Quantitatively measure your DNA

Another perspective provided by science includes the concept of the genome, which refers to your complete genetic blueprint, or DNA. The exposome, on the other hand, encompasses the cumulative effects of all external exposures—such as diet, lifestyle, toxins, and stress—that influence gene expression, primarily through epigenetics. This factor plays a significant role in determining approximately 90 percent of diseases and the aging process. A gene is defined as a specific DNA sequence responsible for coding a particular protein. In summary, the genome represents an individual's entire genetic makeup, while the immunome consists of the genes and proteins that make up the immune system.

In relation to DNA and exosomes in Eastern medicine, there exists an energy cycle that undergoes shifts every ten years. Additionally, celestial changes occur every five years, along with an earthly energy cycle that operates within that same five-year timeframe.

Here are five elementary theory regarding the genome, which serves as your complete genetic blueprint, determined by the DNA inherited from your parents at birth. The exposome encompasses the cumulative effects of all external factors influencing gene expression. It operates on a cycle of ten years, consisting of five-year heavenly and earthly cycles.

Furthermore, while your DNA blueprint is influenced by your birth date, each five-year cycle is dynamic and subject to variation

I did it measure quantitively way by birthday

According the book *The secret language of Birthdays" by Gary Goldschneider said symbolism derived from the configuration of the heavenly constellations with 12 signs.

All the natural rhythms of nature and certain types 5 elements of people should be born at certain times of the years I like the new version of the 5 elementary theory makes it simple and easy to apply to treat patients by patient birthday

birthday is the secret language as wired to universe energy as we were born so I calculate each 5-organ energy dynamic meaning how 5-organ energy distribute and which organ energy is excess or deficiency causing disease

The best model is each 5 organ had an equal amount of energy but most case is biased and unbalanced

This is a unique model that challenges the unclear and vague 5E theory.

Based on the Huang Di Nei Jing, a Eastern medical Bible "Giving a purpose to everything that exists in the universe. The principle that moves all things. Heaven gave me the principle of harmony as my nature, and following my nature is the Way.

There are 3 case of pattern differentiation in chapter 1. I will show you how it works

1 heart energy > lung energy

Firstly, as I mentioned chapter 1 page 32 jane case experienced difficulty breathing, an excess of Fire Access indicates that the heart is overactive and is invading the lungs, resulting in breathing issue see the jane 5 organ energy allocation.

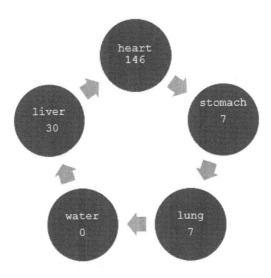

2. heart energy < lung energy

Secondly, page 38 Jenny case an excess of Metal indicates that the fire element is underactive, leading to a runny nose and increased susceptibility to the flu.

See the jenny 5 organ energy allocation

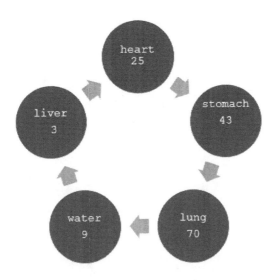

3. heart energy = lung energy

Finally, Page 35 john lung and heart balance case see the john 5 organ energy allocation

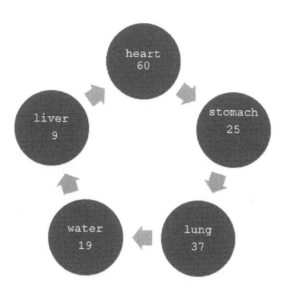

Through simulation, we can determine the energy levels of each of the organs involved.

Although the symptoms may be similar, the underlying causes differ, necessitating different treatment approaches.

For the patient with excess heat, I would recommend cupping therapy to reduce the heat.

Conversely, for the other patient, the goal would be to elevate the heat energy.

The core value of this book lies in understanding the balance of organ-related gene energy. It emphasizes identifying the root causes of health issues and developing long-term treatment plans for disease prevention.

By assessing which organs are overactive and which are underactive, you can create a straightforward plan. This involves nourishing the weaker organs while employing techniques, such as applying heat to underactive organ

Reference

Buteyko Breathing: Six-month Respiratory Medicine training to slow down the breath rate and increase awareness of dysfunctional breathing.

"Lymph and Longevity" by Gerald M. Lenore

"Breath Taking" by Michael J. Stepen, MD.

"Your Brain Explained" by Marc Dingman, PhD

"Circadian Code" by Dr. Satchan.

"The Energy Paradox: What to do when your get up and go has got up and gone" by Steven R. Gundry, MD.

"Drop Acid" by David Perlmutter, MD with Kristin Loberg

"Medical Medium" by Anthony William.

"Young Forever" by Mark Hyman, MD and "Breath: The New Science of a Lost Art" by James Nestor.

"Lifespan" by David A. Sinclair

"Breaking Free from Long Covid" by Dr. Lucy Gahan.

"Be Here Now: Journey of Awakening by Ram Dass"

"The Complete Book of Running" by James E. Fixx

"Doing and Being" by Barnet Bain.

"Infectious Pathogens and How We Fight Them" by Dr. John S. Tregoning

"Time and Medicine" by Larry Dossey, MD

"Beyond Illness: Discovering the Experience of Health" Larry Dossey's

"Pain: Why It Hurts Where It Hurts When It Hurts". Richard Stiller's

"The Aquarian Conspiracy" by Marilyn Ferguson

"The Oxygen Advantage" by Patrick McKeown,

"The Healing Power of the Breath" by Dr. Gerberg and Dr. Brown.

"Let Every Breath" by Vladimir Vasiliev

"The Book of Doing and Being" by Barnet Bain

"Be Here Now: Journey of Awakening" by Ram Dass Leriche,

About the Author

Almost 50 years ago, I was in a terrible car accident at the age of 11. I was crying and wanted to go home I still have clear memories of that day like it was yesterday.

As I progressed, I developed respiratory issues along with heart palpitations and mostly took pills for a runny nose.

After graduating major in economics, I worked for a leading investment company, trading stocks and bonds with IPOs. It was a great time, 10 years of knowing the whole market, researching and analyzing, and dealing with the stress of performance while drinking and smoking.

Slowly, I began to experience health issues, including brain fog and concentration issues, feeling extremely tired.

After having my first baby at the age of 32, I completely collapsed and could not continue with a normal job.

I turned to Eastern medicine school to begin my healing journey.

I was fortunate to meet my mentor, a great sage, in my first class.

he asked me why I was sick, what my constitution was, and explained how my lung organ excess with a deficiency in my heart caused respiratory issues, along with damage to my gut.

This was a eureka moment for me to change my career. Another six years passed quickly as I learned that our body system is like the cosmic system, based on the five elements theory.

After relocating to Canada 30 years ago, I became fascinated by the wonders of Western medical courses, particularly in areas such as anatomy, brain research, and hormonal functions—topics I had never encountered in Eastern medicine. I treated my case of chronic symptoms related to low immunity, including breathing issues that I had been experiencing.

Throughout the pandemic, I dedicated more time to researching the virus and the many lives it has taken. I observed that some treatments are unconventional and that while some patients take medication, they do not address the root causes of their conditions, leading to confusion and a deeper understanding of Western healthcare.

Therefore, I believe it is time to integrate Eastern and Western medicine in addressing the virus, as it is invisible. The scientific data-driven methods of Western medicine combined with the diverse treatment options available in Eastern medicine

I enjoy the podcast by Dr. Mark Hyman, the author of "Forever Young," as well as the website of medical medium William Anthony, the author of "Medical Medium." One of the most inspiring books I've read is "The Wisdom of the Body" by Dr. Walter Bradford Cannon, published in 1930

Printed in the United States
by Baker & Taylor Publisher Services